OBESITY, EATING DISORDERS AND THE MEDIA

Obesity, Eating Disorders and the Media

Edited by

KARIN ELI AND STANLEY ULIJASZEK
University of Oxford, UK

Routledge
Taylor & Francis Group
LONDON AND NEW YORK

First published 2014 by Ashgate Publishing

Published 2016 by Routledge
2 Park Square, Milton Park, Abingdon, Oxon OX14 4RN
711 Third Avenue, New York, NY 10017, USA

Routledge is an imprint of the Taylor & Francis Group, an informa business

British Library Cataloguing in Publication Data
A catalogue record for this book is available from the British Library

The Library of Congress has cataloged the printed edition as follows:
Obesity, eating disorders and the media / [edited] by Karin Eli and Stanley Ulijaszek.
pages cm.
Includes bibliographical references and index.
ISBN 978-1-4094-5771-8 (hardback) 1. Obesity in mass media.
2. Obesity--Social aspects. 3. Eating disorders--Social aspects. 4. Obesity--Social aspects.
I. Karin, Eli, editor of compilation. II. Ulijaszek, Stanley J., editor of compilation.

P96.O23O265 2014
362.196'398--dc23

2014015813

ISBN 9781409457718 (hbk)

Contents

List of Figures, Tables and Boxes

Figure

Tables

Boxes

Notes on Contributors

Rene Almeling's research and teaching interests are at the intersection of gender, medicine and markets. She is the author of the award-winning book, *Sex Cells: The Medical Market for Eggs and Sperm* (University of California Press, 2011). Currently, she is working on several research projects, including a national survey of American attitudes toward genetic risk (with Shana Gadarian), a survey of women's experiences with *in vitro* fertilization, and a new book project on the history of men's health.

Natalie C. Boero is Associate Professor of Sociology at San Jose State University in San Jose, California. She received her PhD in 2006 from the University of California at Berkeley. Her first book, *Killer Fat: Media, Medicine, Morals and the American 'Obesity Epidemic'* was published by Rutgers University Press in 2012.

Michael Davies is a professor, ARC Future Fellow and Co-Director of the Research Centre of Early Origins of Health and Disease at the University of Adelaide. His research in reproductive epidemiology investigates early life factors that impact on the health of Australians within and across generations. He is also researching decision-making, safety and effectiveness of assisted reproductive technologies.

Pino Donghi is Contract Professor at La Sapienza, University of Rome, where he teaches bio-medical communication. Having studied semiotics and theory of communication, he spent the last 25 years researching and working in science communication. From 1994 to 2010, he directed the Fondazione Sigma-tau, organizing 'Spoletoscienza' meetings during the Spoleto Two World Festival. He has also worked together with M° Luca Ronconi and Professor John D. Barrow on staging the 2002 UBU award-winning play *Infinities* at the Piccolo Teatro di Milano. Among other books, he published *Sui Generis* (2006), a collection of essays on the popularization of science. More recently, working as consultant for the Laterza publishing company, he became the editor of Italian cultural festival texts, including the Economy Festival in Trento and the Law Festival in Piacenza.

Karin Eli is a postdoctoral fellow at the University of Oxford's Institute of Social and Cultural Anthropology, where her research focuses on the subjective experience of eating disorders. She has conducted extensive narrative-based research among people with eating disorders in Israel and the UK, and has also collaborated with choreographer Rosie Kay on a project exploring the embodiment of eating disorders through dance practice. As part of the Oxford Food Governance Group, she is currently working on a research project that examines consumer engagement with information and communication technologies (ICT) as an emerging mode of food governance.

Anna Lavis is a medical anthropologist and postdoctoral research fellow at the University of Birmingham. In the multidisciplinary context of the Department of Primary Care, she leads applied research studies into psychosis and eating disorders. Also focused on individuals' lived experiences of mental illness, Anna's doctorate explored pro-anorexia and she continues to publish on eating, eating disorders and bodily materialities. Anna has recently co-edited *Why We Eat, How We Eat: Contemporary Encounters between Foods and Bodies* (Abbots & Lavis, Ashgate 2013) and *Careful Eating: Embodied Entanglements between Food and Care* (Abbots, Lavis & Attala, Ashgate, forthcoming).

Vivienne Moore is a professor and (with Michael Davies) is Co-Director of the Life Course and Intergenerational Health Research Group at the University of Adelaide, South Australia. Her research investigates the social and behavioural influences on women's and children's health within a life-course perspective, and gender inequalities in health.

Abigail C. Saguy is Associate Professor of Sociology and Women's Studies at UCLA. She received a PhD from Princeton University and from the École des Hautes Études en Sciences Sociales (France). She was a Robert Wood Johnson Scholar in Health Policy Research and a fellow at the Center for Advanced Studies in the Behavioral Sciences at Stanford University. She is the author of *What is Sexual Harassment? From Capitol Hill to the Sorbonne* (2003), *What's Wrong with Fat?* (2013), and over 20 articles published in peer-reviewed journals.

Clive Seale is Professor of Sociology at Brunel University. He has written a book about the mass media and health (*Media and Health*, Sage 2002) and occasionally does studies of the way in which the mass media represents particular health topics. His other research concerns end-of-life care and communication in health care settings.

Emily Shepherd graduated in 2010 with an MBBS from Barts and The London School of Medicine, where she completed a B Med Sci in Community Health with First-class honours. Her thesis analysed the representation of eating disorders in newspapers. She has now embarked on a career in obstetrics and gynaecology and is a specialty trainee in North West London.

Helene A. Shugart is a professor in the Department of Communication at the University of Utah. Her expertise lies at the intersection of rhetorical, media and cultural studies. Her most recent work examines public discourses about health and how they are produced, negotiated and circulated in cultural, political and economic context. She is the author (with C.E. Waggoner) of *Making Camp* (2008), and of over 25 peer-reviewed journal articles.

Stanley Ulijaszek is Professor of Human Ecology and Director of both the Unit for Biocultural Variation and Obesity and the Institute of Social and Cultural Anthropology, at the University of Oxford. He is associate editor of *Homo: Journal of Comparative Human Biology*. Among his books are *Nutritional Anthropology* (Smith-Gordon, 1993, with S.S. Strickland), *Human Energetics in Biological Anthropology* (Cambridge University Press, 1995), *Cambridge Encyclopedia of Human Growth and Development* (Cambridge University Press, 1998, with F.E. Johnston and M.A. Preece), *Holistic Anthropology* (Berghahn Books, 2007, with D. Parkin), *Human Variation: From Laboratory to Field* (Cambridge University Press, 2010, with C.G.N. Mascie-Taylor and A. Yasukouchi) and *Evolving Human Nutrition* (Cambridge University Press, 2012, with S. Elton and N. Mann).

Megan Warin is a social anthropologist and Associate Professor in the Discipline of Gender Studies and Social Analysis at the University of Adelaide. Her current research interests span theories of embodiment and new materialisms, intersections of class and gender in experiences of obesity, public understanding of obesity science, and desire and denial in eating disorders.

Josephine Wennerholm holds a BA in child psychology and semiotics. She has worked for the United Nations Food and Agriculture Organization (FAO) as a communications consultant and writer. Based in Rome, Josephine is the European director of a company representing Italian artisans internationally, and continues to pursue her interest in food as a professional cooking teacher.

Tanya Zivkovic is a social anthropologist whose research explores notions of the body and cultural trajectories of the life course. These are themes in her work on death and dying; ethnomedicine, and the intersections of gender, class and obesity. Tanya is a research fellow in the Discipline of Gender Studies and Social Analysis, University of Adelaide.

Preface

Media stories about obesity and eating disorders often create images that bear little resemblance to the scientific, clinical, and even lived realities of these conditions. The result is confusion and contradiction: what is the public to believe about obesity and eating disorders? And *who* should the public believe? For some critics, a frequent suspicion is that the blame lies solely with the messenger – that is, the media themselves – in misrepresenting and reducing complex conditions. With framings that seem to stereotype and stigmatize people with obesity or eating disorders, while simplifying and sometimes misinterpreting scientific research, this suspicion might seem like a foregone conclusion. Yet, as the chapters in this volume demonstrate, media framings are dynamically entangled with the societal, scientific, and political contexts in which they operate. Drawing on interdisciplinary analyses of a range of media – including print and television, news and entertainment – this volume critically examines media framings of obesity and eating disorders as they implicate wider societal anxieties about fat, eating, and disorder, and as they reflect and respond to scientific discourses and policy interests. Throughout the volume, several disconnects emerge between science and media, media and policy, and policy and practice, suggesting that problematic media framings reflect, at least in part, miscommunications and misalignments between the actors who form the contentious, disparate, and complex field of obesity and eating disorders.

This volume developed out of a one-day workshop titled 'Obesity, Eating Disorders, and the Media', which took place at St Anne's College, Oxford, on 9 November 2011. The workshop was convened under the auspices of the University of Oxford's Unit for Biocultural Variation and Obesity. We thank all presenters, as well as discussants Stella Bruzzi (Warwick University), Tanja Schneider (University of Oxford), and Annamaria Carusi (University of Copenhagen), and co-convener David Zeitlyn (University of Oxford), for their insights and contributions. We also thank Amy McLennan, Marisa Macari, Tess Bird, Ynhi Thai, and Maddie Tye for their enthusiastic and efficient coordination of the everyday aspects of the workshop. Above all, we thank the generous spirit in which attendees entered and engaged with the debate, and the BUPA Foundation whose funding made the workshop possible.

This volume, like the workshop that preceded it, not only brings entanglements of science, media, policy, and practice to the foreground, but also strikes a note of pragmatism. Vivienne Parry, a virtual presenter at the workshop, spoke up for a pragmatic approach. She argued that, to maximize impact, the scientific community must present the media with practical, authority-questioning, clearly achievable research recommendations that promise a quick win. Yet the workings of this formula continue to elude scholars and scientists. To understand what the media might construe as 'practical', 'authoritative', and 'achievable' obesity and eating disorders research recommendations, we must first understand the lenses through which media frame these conditions. Through illuminating the logics that underlie media representations of obesity and eating disorders, scientists and policy makers alike will be better positioned to challenge the status-quo. We hope that this volume will contribute to, and indeed increase, the capacity to bring about change.

Karin Eli and Stanley Ulijaszek
Oxford, UK
June 2014

Chapter 1
Introduction: Obesity, Eating Disorders and the Media

Karin Eli and Stanley Ulijaszek

This volume is premised on the idea that we can best understand the media's representations of obesity and eating disorders by conceptualizing them as closely interlinked, rather than distinct, public health and social phenomena. It questions the tendency to position the obese and the anorexic body as separate, polar opposites – as overeating juxtaposed with self-starvation. Instead, this volume approaches obesity and eating disorders as mutually-implicating conditions that together draw attention to the material extremes of fat and emaciated bodies, overeating and self-starvation, and fatty and lean foods.

Eating disorders and obesity are not, in themselves, contrasting conditions. While obesity can be defined by *metrics*, such as body mass index, eating disorders are defined primarily through *ideation* and *practice*; underweight, rather than being the endpoint of eating disorders, is only one possible outcome. Far from being mutually exclusive, obesity and eating disorders, at times, co-exist, and the clinical literature has long recognized connections between the two conditions. As early as the 1970s, prominent eating disorders clinicians such as Hilde Bruch (1974) and Arthur Crisp (1980) published case study monographs that highlighted links between obesity and eating disorders, and implicated childhood obesity as a risk factor for the development of anorexia nervosa later in life. The newly published fifth edition of the *Diagnostic and Statistical Manual* (*DSM-V*) (American Psychiatric Association, 2013) recognizes binge eating disorder – which often leads to obesity – as one of the three specified eating disorders, alongside anorexia nervosa and bulimia nervosa. Moreover, boundaries between the three eating disorders (and their subclinical variants, subsumed under other specified feeding or eating disorder [OSFED]), are highly fluid. While it may appear that binge eating disorder and anorexia nervosa entail significantly different eating practices, anorexia nervosa does have a binge eating and purging subtype, and most people with eating disorders, including those diagnosed with anorexia nervosa, have binge eating experiences during the course of their disorder (Fairburn and Harrison, 2003). And rather than remaining fixed in their diagnoses, people with eating disorders, particularly those initially diagnosed with restrictive anorexia nervosa, may transition from one diagnosis to another (Eddy et al., 2002; Eddy et al., 2008). Indeed, Fairburn, Cooper and Shafran (2003) argue that a 'transdiagnostic' approach to understanding and treating eating disorders best reflects the cognitive realities of these disorders.

For the lay public, however, clinically-observed connections between obesity and eating disorders are not readily apparent. Popular imaginings of obesity and eating disorders tend to relegate these conditions to contrasting points on the continuum of body weight. Yet this misperception also links obesity and eating disorders through their seeming disparity. In lay framings of obesity and eating disorders, the two conditions are submerged in inescapable co-existence, not within the same *person*, but within the same *society*. Whether explicitly or implicitly, lay framings of one condition vis-à-vis its 'other' reveal a form of cultural 'sense-making' that interweaves the construction of social problems, a fascination with the body in extremes, and the zeitgeist of normative body image and consumption concerns in the twenty-first century.

Bridging the clinical and lay realms are the news media. In recent years, the news media landscape has been undergoing rapid change with the emergence of influential new media and social media platforms, enabling more local control and user involvement. Amidst these changes, the media ('traditional' and new) continue to be the central source of research information for the public, while also providing the main platform for lay (albeit, at times, journalistically-mediated) discussion, dissemination, and consumption of dominant popular ideas on obesity and eating disorders. The news media, importantly, broker knowledge, making visible selected scientific findings and policy decisions, while leaving many others obscured: even to the well-versed lay reader, most scientific and policy papers remain inaccessible, such that the public – beyond certain academic and government circles – must rely on news media to learn about scientific and policy work. Analyses of media framings of obesity and eating disorders, then, can unveil two central constituents of popular 'sense-making': how lay discourses constitute these conditions as social problems, and how scientific and policy news is transmitted to the public.

To develop a new, interlinked perspective on media representations of obesity and eating disorders, we set out to delineate the themes underlying media framings of these conditions, and elucidate the news media's selective coverage and representation of scientific and policy reports. Reflecting these dual aims, this volume is divided into two sections: 'Rhetorics of abjection and alarm' and 'Representations of science and policy'. We suggest that richer understandings emerge when media representations of obesity and media representations of eating disorders – and of the bodies attendant to each of these conditions – are read together. Such reading provides fertile ground from which to explore the discursive parallels these representations share, consider how the framing of one condition implicates the other, and examine how these framings reflect the greater socio-political space within which obesity and eating disorders, and the science and policy thereof, occur.

The book begins with Anna Lavis' analysis of the morally-condemning media discourses surrounding pro-anorexia websites. Lavis examines the ways in which these discourses have become entangled in the (re)production of pro-anorexia (pro-ana) online, their reductionist, and indeed, judgmental framings of pro-ana redefining pro-anorexic cyber spaces as zones of (malicious) contagion. These media stories, Lavis argues, have practical bearing on the sites and people they frame, as they facilitate, even encourage, engagements that overtake and transform pro-anorexic spaces. Media tales of anorexic 'contagion' online facilitate and legitimize interlopers – 'righteously indignant' outsiders, and those seeking to be 'infected' – whose entry into pro-anorexic spaces then reinforces the media's reductionist framing of pro-ana as a cause for alarm. The framing of pro-ana through an alarmist lens is, perhaps, not surprising; even predating the pro-ana era, media stories have portrayed eating disorders as 'infectious', preying on women's supposedly inherent vulnerabilities (to images, texts, and other women), and being transmitted from one 'victim' to another through, paradoxically, the media themselves (cf. Bray, 1996; Burke, 2006). But alarmist media framings are not restricted to presumed social contagion. As Natalie C. Boero suggests in her chapter on *New York Times* articles, the news media frame the 'obesity epidemic' as an impending nation-wide public health crisis brought on by irresponsible, ill-educated, or self-indulgent eating and (non-)exercise behaviours. While media reports on obesity sound the alarm for a population much broader than the teenage girls identified in reports on pro-ana, the crisis they portray is also bound up with groups they identify as being 'susceptible', particularly women and ethnic minority citizens of reduced or deprived means. Borrowing the language of epidemiology, media reports dissect these groups' socio-environmental realities into practices that equal vulnerability and risk, reducing them into variables that do not reflect people's own lived experience. And much like media stories on pro-ana, media reports then frame these 'at risk' groups as posing risk to wider society.

Alarm is central in media framings of both obesity and eating disorders; yet, when media portrayals of people with eating disorders and people with obesity are considered together, suggestive differences in the styles of alarm emerge. In their comparative analysis of media stories on people with eating disorders and people with obesity, Saguy and Gruys (2010) pointed to the intersectionality of gender, race, and class in the moral framings of these stories. Eating disordered women, they argued, were framed sympathetically, their white, middle class status affording the protective labelling of disease 'victim', in sharp contrast to the moral condemnation levelled at the often non-white, working class or poor people with obesity portrayed in media stories as bearing responsibility for their condition. As Ferris (2003) suggested in her analysis of media stories on Carnie Wilson and Tracey Gold (US celebrity women known for their obesity and anorexia, respectively), while media stories situate both obese and anorexic people at the margins of society, they frame them at odds: the latter as afflicted and in need of re-incorporation, and the former as blame-worthy and requiring ostracism.

In this volume, however, we expand the comparative discussion beyond the realm of biomedically defined disorders, and toward an exploration of the murkier ground occupied by the 'extreme' bodies these disorders connote. The obese body and the emaciated body do not simply connote disorder; they are suffused with the materiality of fat, muscle, and bones, and the discourses thereof. It is this materiality that Pino Donghi and Josephine Wennerholm explore in their chapter on the moral dimensions of fat in popular media images and texts. Donghi and Wennerholm draw parallels between media framings of bodies and foods, arguing that both are imagined through similar aesthetic and moral lenses. Fat, especially, looms large. Christopher Forth (2013) argues that stereotypes of fat as morally transgressive or abject are associated, historically, with responses to the sensory properties of fat, its slipperiness and softness. In Donghi and Wennerholm's analysis, fat emerges as a substance that, as framed by contemporary media stories, pervades both indulgent foods and indolent bodies, implicating failure to embody the self-controlled ethic of neoliberal citizenship. Lean foods and lean bodies, on the other hand, are portrayed in the media as embodying the streamlined, minimalist aesthetic of this political era.

In their material being, the emaciated body and the fat body, moreover, implicate one another. The imagining of the emaciated body in juxtaposition to, and intimate linking with, the obese body has historical roots that extend further than the biomedical and epidemiological definitions of obesity and eating disorders. The situating of fat and wasted bodies as objects for public display can be traced back through the cultural history of enfreakment and spectacle, where 'living skeletons', 'fat men', and 'fat ladies' were stock characters in the travelling menageries of the freak show carnival; as Thomson (1996) writes, 'living skeletons' and 'fat ladies' were often theatrically coupled, positioned on stage one next to the other to enhance their individual 'extreme'. Yet seemingly egalitarian exaggerations of 'extremeness' do not carry the same implications for the bodies they contrast. In their chapter on the visceral and moral worlds of UK reality show 'Supersize vs. Superskinny', Karin Eli and Anna Lavis demonstrate how the show's direct juxtaposition of fat and skinny bodies constructs the fat body as abject, dangerous, and in need of education and reform. Eli and Lavis argue that the show, which brings together obese and underweight participants who then eat each other's meals, evokes disgust – directed at both fatty foods and fat bodies – to develop a tacit learning of abjection. In portraying fat as abject, and teaching participants to regard their chosen foods, and their own bodies, as such, the show frames abjection as a central element of public health education – as the sensation all must embody, in reaction to fat, if society is to reverse the alarmingly increasing rates of population obesity.

Abjection and alarm, however, are not confined to reality show, magazine, and newspaper feature framings of obesity and eating disorders. As the book's second section shows, these framings also shape news media reports on science and policy concerning these conditions. We begin this section with Megan Warin, Tanya Zivkovic, Vivienne Moore and Michael Davies' chapter on media representations of the fetal origins hypothesis as applied to obesity. As the authors argue, while the hypothesis implicates socio-environmental variables in the development of obesity, its representations cite women (particularly those living in poverty) as the causal agents shaping adverse uterine environments, and thereby transmitting obesity to the next generation. It becomes apparent, then, that while media reports on the fetal origins hypothesis may purport to explain a complex scientific concept to the public, they reproduce judgmental constructions of gender, race, and class, made 'objective' through the (mis)use of scientific research. Emily Martin (1991; 1994) has argued that bioscientific representations of physiological phenomena are themselves inflected with implicit social, political, and gendered constructions. Yet, as Warin et al. show in their chapter, news media framings may even distort the representation of a phenomenon in order to shape the story for a socially recognized template of alarm.

The familiar framings of abjection and alarm offer a way of simplifying the biomedical and environmental complexities associated with obesity and eating disorders. In their analysis of US newspaper coverage of eating disorder stories, O'Hara and Clegg Smith (2007) found that most articles employed simplistic, alarmist framings, reducing the medical complexity of eating disorders to support a journalistic entertainment agenda. Emily Shepherd and Clive Seale suggest in their comparative analysis of UK and US media coverage of eating disorders that the extent of reductionism and sensationalism may be dependent on the news source: the character of news media reports on eating disorders, they found, varies by nation and the intellectual standing of the media source. Yet, Shepherd and Seale argue that entertainment-centred framings – mainly focused on portrayals of (rumoured) celebrity illness– constitute the main template by which popular newspapers provide information, and even education, on eating disorders to the widest segment of the lay public. Familiar templates, however, not only affect the ways in which scientific findings are reported; they may also affect *which* scientific findings are reported. In their chapter on scientific reports concerning obesity, their attendant press releases, and the media coverage that followed, Abigail Saguy and Rene Almeling find that media reports employ alarmist framings to convey scientific findings. Saguy and Almeling suggest, moreover, that the news media may actively choose to report on those research findings that best fit an alarmist frame. Yet they also note that media reports make use of another facilitator of simplified reporting – the press release. Issued by the *Journal of the American Medical Association*, the press releases the authors studied employed alarmist framings similar to those later included in the media reports. It is possible, then, that press releases may operate symbiotically with news media reports, creating a positive feedback loop: to ensure the popular dissemination of biomedical research findings, press releases employ familiar framings, accessible to the public; journalists then deploy these framings in news media reports; and the reappearance of these framings in the popular news media further reinforces their cultural import.

The news media's familiar templates of representation also hold sway in the reporting of policy discussions concerning obesity and eating disorders: influence which, in turn, can have consequences in practice. Examining news media coverage of UK obesity policy reports, Stanley Ulijaszek finds that media coverage tends to reduce complex reports on public health policies, with alarmist and individual-centred framings guiding the simplification process. Ulijaszek suggests that, in so doing, media sources re-engage with pre-set parameters for evaluating obesity, thereby providing a selective, often critical view of obesity policy that may reinforce stasis, rather than action. And, closing the book, Helene A. Shugart's systematic analysis of obesity coverage in leading US media sources suggests that a persistent mismatch characterizes the relationship between media and policy framings of obesity. The public, Shugart argues, is exposed to multiple popular framings of obesity in the media, yet none of these framings is compatible with the discourses employed in public health efforts. This incompatibility, according to Shugart, may explain the ineffectiveness of obesity prevention policies to date. As the chapters by Ulijaszek and Shugart suggest, science and policy stories that fall outside known narrative templates, or that outright challenge them, may not reach the public. Health policy, when communicated to and distilled for the public, must participate in a lay public process of sense-making and fit a known template, in order to be selected for dissemination and effectively conveyed.

Together, the chapters that comprise this volume provoke critical reflection on the ways in which media framings of obesity and eating disorders might express and influence public perceptions of these conditions, as well as the policies that concern them. Exploring the news media's uses of abjection and alarm, simplification and reduction, and the rationales therein, this volume brings to the foreground processes of sense-making that often remain hidden from view. As new media continue to increase in variety, dissemination, and influence, and with the interest in obesity and eating disorders – alongside the bodies and food practices they implicate – showing no signs of abating, we hope this volume will inspire future research on how these themes and processes might underlie media framings.

References

American Psychiatric Association. Task Force on DSM-V. (2013). *Diagnostic and statistical manual of mental disorders: DSM-V*. Amer Psychiatric Pub Inc.

Bray, A. (1996). The anorexic body: Reading disorders. *Cultural Studies, 10(3)*, 413–429.

Bruch, H. (1974). *Eating disorders: Obesity, anorexia nervosa, and the person within*. London: Routledge and Kegan Paul.

Burke, E. (2006). Feminine visions: Anorexia and contagion in pop discourse. *Feminist Media Studies, 6(3)*, 315–330.

Crisp, A.H. (1980). *Anorexia nervosa: Let me be*. London: Academic Press.

Eddy, K.T., Keel, P.K., Dorer, D.J., et al. (2002). Longitudinal comparison of anorexia nervosa subtypes. *International Journal of Eating Disorders, 31(2)*, 191–201.

Eddy, K.T., Dorer, D.J., Franko, D.L., et al. (2008). Diagnostic crossover in anorexia nervosa and bulimia nervosa: Implications for DSM-V. *The American Journal of Psychiatry, 165(2)*, 245.

Fairburn, C.G. & Harrison, P.J. (2003). Eating disorders. *The Lancet, 361(9355)*, 407–416.

Fairburn, C.G., Cooper, Z. & Shafran, R. (2003). Cognitive behaviour therapy for eating disorders: A 'transdiagnostic' theory and treatment. *Behaviour Research and Therapy, 41(5)*, 509–528.

Ferris, J.E. (2003). Parallel discourses and 'appropriate' bodies: Media constructions of anorexia and obesity in the cases of Tracey Gold and Carnie Wilson. *Journal of Communication Inquiry, 27(3)*, 256–273.

Forth, C.E. (2013). The qualities of fat: Bodies, history, and materiality. *Journal of Material Culture, 18(2)*, 135–154.

Martin, E. (1991). The egg and the sperm: How science has constructed a romance based on stereotypical male-female roles. *Signs, 16(3)*, 485–501.

Martin, E. (1994). *Flexible bodies: Tracking immunity in American culture from the days of polio to the age of AIDS*. Boston: Beacon Press.

O'Hara, S.K. & Smith, K.C. (2007). Presentation of eating disorders in the news media: What are the implications for patient diagnosis and treatment? *Patient Education and Counseling, 68(1)*, 43–51.

Saguy, A.C. & Gruys, K. (2010). Morality and health: News media constructions of overweight and eating disorders. *Social Problems, 57(2)*, 231–250.

Thomson, R.G. (1996). Introduction: From wonder to error – a genealogy of freak discourse in modernity. In R.G. Thomson (ed.), *Freakery: Cultural spectacles of the extraordinary body* (pp. 1–19). New York: New York University Press.

PART I
Rhetorics of Abjection and Alarm

In this section, we examine media representations of obesity and eating disorders as linked through rhetorical abjection and alarm, both textual and visual. Through these twin lenses, we explore how the media position obesity and eating disorders along a thematic axis, as threatening, mutually-implicating conditions of 'extreme' bodies, foods, and eating practices. The section begins with Anna Lavis' analysis of the morally-condemning media discourses surrounding pro-anorexia websites, and how these discourses have become entangled in the (re)production of pro-anorexia online. Discourses of individual blame also feature centrally in Natalie Boero's analysis of the 'obesity epidemic' as portrayed in *The New York Times*, where she highlights discursive intersections of gender, class, race, moral behaviour, and public health risk. Exploring moral dimensions of fat in popular media images and texts, Pino Donghi and Josephine Wennerholm draw links between media framings of food and the body, suggesting that media imaginings equate lean foods and lean bodies with similar moral and aesthetic typologies, both representing an idealized 'self-control', while fat is equated with turpitude, impurity, and desire. Finally, Karin Eli and Anna Lavis explore the visceral and moral worlds of the UK reality show 'Supersize vs. Superskinny', where, they argue, the participants' tacit learning of abjection – vis-à-vis both fatty foods and fat bodies – is constructed as central to the prevention and reversal of obesity.

Chapter 2
Alarming Engagements? Exploring Pro-Anorexia Websites in/and the Media

Anna Lavis

Anorexia's got nothing to do with my body.
The physical bit's just a symptom of my mind.
Eva – inpatient

Introduction

In our online interview, Aurelie,[1] who has created and participated in a number of pro-anorexia websites since the year 2000, offered me their history:

> The very first one was started by a person whose screen name was Empressanorexia_nyc.[2] She started the group on Yahoo called Anorexia with Pride (AWP). It is unknown how, at that time period, many other folks came across it and decided to start their own. It expanded to other various hosts (i.e. MSN, Excite, E-groups) until attention was brought to it from other eating disorder recovery sites. Soon, the webhosts of those sites started banning and deleting any clubs and groups.

Originating in listservs in the mid-1990s before technological advances gave rise to more sophisticated cyber-spaces, pro-anorexia websites were initially created by participants to online eating disorder recovery groups who desired spaces focused more on experiences of illness than the promotion of recovery. As such, variously referred to as 'pro-ana' or 'proana', pro-anorexia websites are, most simply speaking, established and participated in by individuals living with eating disorders. Since the late twentieth century, these sites have generated a plethora of words across print media, television and cyberspace. They have also featured in fiction (Ellis, 2012; Halse Anderson, 2009) and memoirs of

1 All names are research pseudonyms unless stated otherwise.

2 Although Empressanorexia_nyc is cited by Aurelie as their originator, data on the founders of the earliest pro-anorexia website/listserv varies, with other possibilities being 'Narcissa', 'DietPepsiUhHuh' and 'Catarina'. Many thanks to AnaGirlEmpath (not a research pseudonym) for clarifications regarding the history of pro-anorexia websites.

anorexia (Mikhaylenko, 2012), as well as engendering both academic and popular discussions (see Black, 2012; Uca, 2004). However, despite the ebb and flow of their visibility across these diverse moments of 'public culture' (Ortner, 2006) and the media imaginings that coalesce around them, definitions of pro-anorexia websites vary. *Urban Dictionary* defines them as 'a type of website that promotes anorexia' and their participants as 'someone who thinks anorexia is a lifestyle and gets help from a web community to achieve his/her goals'.[3] A recent academic study has likewise argued that they 'encourage knowledge, attitudes, and behaviours to achieve terribly low body weights' (Borzekowski et al., 2010: 1526). Yet, on the homepage of a pro-anorexia website the creator writes that this is 'a place where people with eating disorders can distribute advice and support without censorship', and this aspect of support has also been highlighted in academic analyses. Although nominally pro-*anorexic* – with anorexia as the diagnosis around which most discussions and desires coalesce – to the sites there is a definitional fluidity; participants may have diagnoses of – and seek support for – anorexia nervosa, bulimia nervosa, EDNOS[4] and may also transition between these during the time in which they engage with these websites. Mirroring this heterogeneity of definition and diagnostic fluidity, it is unclear how many pro-anorexia websites there are. A recent estimate put their number at 400–500 (Bond, 2012) but, as Aurelie states above, beginning with *Yahoo's* response to the first media discussions of pro-anorexia in *The Salon* magazine (Brown, 2001) and by Oprah Winfrey, since 2001 the large global servers have shut down websites making any references to pro-anorexia (see also Reaves, 2001). This has led the sites to continually reappear in different guises or make themselves more hidden. Pro-anorexia websites have historically shared certain key elements, which are: discussion forums; food avoidance advice, known as *Tips & Tricks*; journal entries; clinical information about anorexia, bulimia and EDNOS, often taken from the DSM-IV (APA, 1994) and *Thinspiration*, which consists of photographs of starving bodies and, sometimes, celebrities. However, these features are no longer the sole domain of pro-anorexia websites; they also leak into the wider landscape of the Internet. Since it became a public site in 2006, *Facebook* has seen an emergence of groups calling themselves pro-anorexic, and these have been subject to enforced closure by the site's administrators. *Tumblr, Instagram* and *Pinterest* also witnessed a wave of content terming itself pro-anorexic, which led to all three to ban this in early 2012 (Barnett, August 2012; *Daily Mail*, unattributed, March 26, 2012). Or rather, we might say that they banned what they *regarded* as pro-anorexia but, crucially, this is not as simple as it might seem. When tropes that are traditionally part of pro-anorexia websites, such as *Thinspiration*, appear in other cyber spaces, they accrue and transmit very different meanings from those they have on the websites. On pro-anorexia websites themselves, moreover, there

3 http://www.urbandictionary.com/define.php?term=pro+ana [accessed 8 March 2013].

4 Eating Disorder Not Otherwise Specified.

is also now an increasing multiplicity to their meanings. What 'counts' as pro-anorexia – and indeed is counted in determining the number of the websites – varies according to the imaginings of pro-anorexia, and indeed of anorexia itself, that are being drawn on. Despite the perpetually-changing, multivocal nature of the Internet, this heterogeneity cannot be attributed only to the medium itself. Rather, it highlights what it is that requires exploration about the relationships that exist between pro-anorexia websites and the media coverage that frames and, even, performs them.

Therefore, to explore these websites in/and the media, this chapter draws on a selection of social and news media from early reports in 2001 to more recent ones in 2013, alongside data from anthropological observations and interviews on pro-anorexia websites (2005–2013) and in an English eating disorders inpatient clinic (2007–2008). Whilst being careful not to unthinkingly transfer meanings between diverging spaces of social action, these ethnographic data are employed to respond to a recent suggestion that 'little is known about why people use [pro-anorexia websites]' (Bond, 2012); by contextualizing website participants' online practices in wider articulations of anorexia as 'valued and visible' (Schmidt & Treasure, 2006), the data offer an alternative portrait of pro-anorexia websites to those most often found in the media. Yet, these diverging ways of seeing the sites are not presented only as tales of binary opposition. Rather, holding participants' voices in the same analytical space as media coverage elucidates how the media are *part of* the story of these sites; it reveals their role in the interactive processes through which 'pro-anorexia' has been fractured, multiplied, but also fixed by the words that mire it in controversy.

Traversing a layered textual, virtual and actual landscape in analysis also echoes how participants themselves navigate online and offline worlds; many have been – or, in the case of some of my interviewees, may concomitantly be – in eating disorders treatment. This glimpse into clinical realities also serves, importantly, to remind us that anorexia may be 'dark and dangerous and [leave] a shell of a human being in its wake', as John Evans writes in his memoir (2011: 19). To recognize that anorexia is valued, and even actively maintained, by individuals is not to ignore the distress or ambivalence many feel, and which is also central to pro-anorexia websites. As such, addressing something as complex, intimate and socially taboo as pro-anorexia necessitates acknowledging the extreme danger posed by the illness whilst also taking account of the voices of participants to the sites. This chapter therefore attempts an 'active listening that challenges the listener's preconceptions and positions while at the same time it engages critically with the content of what is being said and heard' (Back, 2007: 23) by individuals who maintain their anorexia on the Internet.

The chapter begins by tracing the alarm present in media coverage of pro-anorexia websites, which views them as populated either by 'victims' or 'predators', before turning to explore the contrasting complexities in participants' own descriptions of why they visit the sites. Participants' accounts elucidate how desire and ambivalence are conjoined as pro-anorexia may signify both a response to, and reconfiguration of, conditions of possibility already compromised by anorexia. Yet it is also in the context of the value placed on this existing illness that we see how, to participants, pro-anorexia websites are not simply about achieving a thin body. Rather, in highlighting a sense of stasis and the importance of 'authentic' diagnosis, they draw our attention to the specific ways that thinness comes to be valued *within* anorexia. Contrasting this to the imaginings of anorexia, bodily thinness and an assumed relationship between these, which underscore much reporting of pro-anorexia websites, illustrates that interactions between the media and the websites are looping rather than linear. The media's words have been active, altering the landscape of the sites and redefining pro-anorexia and even anorexia itself, over the last decade in surprising and, even, harmful ways.

'Predators', 'Victims' and Media Imaginings

During interviews conducted online with participants to pro-anorexia websites, a number of my informants explained that after a spike in media attention, such as that following a press release put out by the UK Eating Disorders Association (now B-eat) in 2006 (Bloomfield, 2006), the pro-anorexia websites in which they participated often had an influx of visitors posting vitriolic hate mail. One such message during fieldwork in 2011 read: 'you dumb idiots I hope you die'. In a slightly more empathetic vein, another visitor wrote, also in 2011:

> This is absolutely sickening! It's one thing to lose weight, but to get so thin that your ribs and bones stick out is just revolting. Guys may flirt with you now, but when they see how sickening you're gonna get they will be scared of you. Oh god, if only you'd listen to someone. You need help!

These messages suggest that the first question we might pose is: what is it about pro-anorexia websites that incites such passionate responses to them? It is arguably not sufficient to propose that the answer lies in their name – that being *pro*-anorexic inherently makes what has been termed 'the dark world of pro-anorexia websites' (Doward & Reilly, 2003) more dangerous than the rest of the seething ambiguity that is cyberspace. Pro-anorexia websites are part of a wider 'medicalization of cyberspace' (Miah & Rich, 2008; see also Gibbon & Novas, 2008), which forged an intimacy between biomedicine and the Internet early in the latter's history. Cyber peer-to-peer interactions among individuals with, especially chronic, health conditions have been widely documented (Fox, 2011; Ziebland & Wyke, 2012) and the re-evaluation of medical knowledge intrinsic to any sense of being *pro*-anorexic is found in those spaces as well as in earlier offline patient groups (cf. Kellener, 1994). It is also now possible to 'find a community to which you can listen or reveal yourself, and instant validation for your condition, whatever it may be' (Elliott, 2004: 217). Hence, there are currently many cyber 'biosocialities' (Rabinow, 1999) around conditions, belief systems and practices also normatively regarded as 'harmful'. Suicide, apotemnophilia (see Elliott, 2004) and self-harm, for example, are all the focus of websites embodying a similarly ambiguous mix of support, 'expertification' (Epstein, 1996), desire and even encouragement. Yet, although these have hit the headlines (cf. Manning, 2012; Townsend, 2013), pro-anorexia websites have incited more media alarm. Thus, perhaps what we really need to ask is: what is it that the media says about pro-anorexia websites that incites vitriolic reactions of the kind noted above?

Media discussions over the last 12 years have commonly dually positioned participants to these websites – as unknowing victims of a disease they do not realize they have or as predators luring others into a 'cult' (Courtney-Smith, 2006) of anorexia within which disease is denied. 'Sick' (Wostear, 2007; also Gotthelf, 2001), 'porn' (Goodchild, 2006), 'macabre' (Doward & Reilly, 2003) and 'revulsion followed by a kind of morbid fascination' (Reaves, 2001) are all descriptions in British newspapers that have fallen into the latter of these poles. Positioning pro-anorexia websites as predatory aligns them with wider cultural and media discussions of the Internet as a dangerous space – even a seductively sexual dangerous space. Labelled as 'literally killing people' (*Daily Mail*, unattributed, 2007), the sites have been called 'sinister online groups' (BBC, unattributed, 2005) focused on the 'promotion of anorexia and competitive dieting' (Laurance, 2012). Justifications for, and illustrations of, this seductive danger are habitually drawn from two particular aspects which are held up as the sites' central features; these are *Tips & Tricks* and *Thinspiration*. I will explore these later in the context of informants' narratives and particular focus will be given to *Thinspiration* as the moment at which website participants' voices and media imaginings encounter one another in generative ways.

Tips & Tricks comprise advice on how to avoid food, forget hunger and hide starvation's physical effects. An example is: 'Spoil your food. As soon as you've cooked your meal, put too much salt, pepper, vinegar, detergent or perfume on it. That way you won't want to eat it'. Referring to such *Tips* a media report, which was part of the surge of interest following the Nominet Trust-funded report into pro-anorexia websites in 2012 (Bond, 2012), stated:

> Worryingly, pro-ana sites do not stop at simply encouraging thinness [...]. They also take an active approach by offering tips on weight loss, dieting and how to maintain an eating disorder, for example, telling readers how to avoid detection from their friends and loved ones. As well as encouraging the use of diet soda, diet pills and cigarettes to suppress the appetite, some pro-ana websites even hold weight loss competitions among their subscribers. (Girtz, 2013)

As this article demonstrates, there has been a prevalent media emphasis on these sites as competitive (cf. Asthana, 2007; Catan & Bennett, 2007; Howard, 2007; Wostear, 2007), replete with 'desire to be the "best anorexic"' (Atkins, 2002). In the UK, *The Independent* recently encapsulated this stance, stating that they encourage: 'young girls to post pictures of their stick-thin bodies to drive one another into losing dangerous amounts of weight in competitive and sometimes startling ways' (*Independent*, unattributed, 2012). Such claims have been accompanied by first-person accounts of being an 'internet anorexic' (Lipinksi, 2007), describing 'group fasts' and 'diet pills, laxatives, diuretics' (ibid. 63). This focus on competition positions pro-anorexia websites not only as spaces that make individuals who already have anorexia more ill, but also that *turn* those without the illness into anorexics, luring them into the entrapment of eating disorders; it is suggested that they 'seduce girls into anorexia' (Levenkron in Dolan, 2003). Such representations resonate with wider media imaginings of mental illness as societally dangerous (Thornicroft, 2006, esp. chapter 6) and, like those depictions of 'feared' or 'deviant' illness, they remind us that 'any disease that is treated as a mystery and acutely enough feared will be felt to be morally, if not literally, contagious' (Sontag, 2002: 3).

Exchanging the words 'disturbing' (Gregoire, September 2012; Morris 2002; Piotrowski, 2013) and 'twisted' (Brown, 2001) for 'disturbed' (Wostear, 2007) and 'troubled' (Doward & Reilly, 2003), the second frequent pole of media representation focuses on unknowing 'victims' who are 'pushed' (BBC, unattributed, 2007) into anorexia – presumably by the 'predators' described above, which splits participants into two distinct groups. Illustrated by a 2007 article in *The Sun,* this depicts the sites as 'a disturbed community of anorexia sufferers who rely on sordid internet information to help them lose weight' (Wostear, 2007). Such coverage echoes wider discussions of the influence of the Internet on behaviour and, in particular, of women as somehow 'intrinsically' more susceptible to media influences than men (see Bell, 2009; Bray, 1996), which also emerge in debates around size zero. As such, this coverage is underpinned by particular assumptions regarding the gender and age make-up of pro-anorexia websites. There is a clear adherence to referring to them as 'aimed at teenage girls' (Atkins, 2002) and to describing the participants in this way (cf. Catan & Bennett, 2007; Driscoll, 2012; Gotthelf, 2001). Yet, whilst the majority of participants are female, some are male. Age, on the other hand, varies widely and the sites are certainly not only visited by adolescents. During their interviews, many informants who were between 30 and 40 years of age recounted visiting pro-anorexia websites every day, sometimes for hours at a time. However, this population tended not to post or upload, their engagements thus leaving no trace. It is their silent participation in the sites that begins to tell us a different story from the media binary highlighted so far. Within that – the framing of 'victims' as becoming ever more anorexic, prey to the encouragement of other participants, and 'predators' as encouraging, and even *turning*, others – there is a sense of movement; seeing pro-anorexia websites as spaces in which to 'achieve' – or produce in others – extreme thinness frames them as teleological. Yet, 'hanging around' on the sites every day, even if not positing, hints at a different temporality; it speaks of stasis, stillness and even entrapment and these are crucial to an understanding of what pro-anorexia websites mean to those who participate in them.

Stasis and Illness: Maintaining Anorexia in Cyberspace

In her online interview, Nancy said of her participation in pro-anorexia websites: 'because we're at a place that already knows tips/tricks, blah blah blah ... we just talk'. This word 'talk' arose in many informants' descriptions of cyber-interactions that encompassed friendship and mutual support. These involved 'discussing things off the telly', as one informant put it, as much as sharing experiences of anorexia. Non-anorexia-focused and anorexia-focused contents thread together on pro-anorexia websites in a 'storied sociality' (Stewart, 1996: 9) and this mix also weaves through their more formalized aspects, such as journals written by the *webmistress/master* (creator) or participants. At times these are 'innocuous, dealing with mundane adolescent concerns' (Giles, 2006: 464). At others, they may be poignant admixtures of pain, pride and both a desire for, and hatred of, anorexia. As such, many informants echoed one participant, Leanne's, words when she argued that pro-anorexia websites are 'not like some evil cult trying to brainwash people into starving themselves it's about giving people support in some of the toughest times of their lives'. Likewise, Laura said: 'I am sick of people talking about how terrible pro ana sites are. In my lowest times I spent endless hours in the chatrooms ... just being happy that there was someone who understood what I was going through and cared if I was sad'. Like Laura, informants described the value of the sites as lying in such understanding and lack of judgement.

That pro-anorexia websites can be 'a sanctuary for those already suffering the illness, a place where they can share their thoughts on anorexia away from the pressure of family or friends who may encourage or enforce recovery' (Burke, 2009: 63–64) has been recognized both in academic analyses (cf. Davies & Lipsey, 2003; Dias, 2003; Pollack, 2003; Wilson et al., 2006; Yeshua-Katz & Martins, 2012) and in some media coverage (Brown, 2001) as far back as the websites' early days. This recognition also lay behind the British Eating Disorders Association's (now B-eat) decision not to back a proposed ban of the sites (see Bloomfield, 2006). However, as a spokeswoman for the US National Eating Disorders Association (NEDA) recently suggested, offering a 'sense of belonging' (Mysko in Gregoire, September 2012) and support to participants also 'validates their experiences' (ibid.). The sharing of affects and desires that is part of the websites' 'storied sociality' (Stewart, 1996) serves to legitimize participants' feelings about anorexia, personhood and relationships between these. Such exchanges can therefore, as the media have argued, deepen existing anorexia. In normalizing the illness, they have the potential to lead participants to not seek other forms of help (see Bardone-Cone & Cass, 2006; Mulveen & Hepworth, 2006; Tierney, 2006; Wilson et al., 2006). This 'negative enabling' (Haas et al., 2011) was recognized by informants during their interviews. In hers, Nora wrote: 'I get both support and motivation if someone is going too far the community would say something but what is too far? If I wanted help I wouldn't be looking up pro ana websites so people who are on those sites want to be supported to continue with the illness'.

This process of normalization has frequently been equated in media coverage with denial of illness, leading to claims that 'pro-ana refers to the rejection of the idea that anorexia nervosa is an eating disorder' (Udovitch, 2002). It is suggested that participants have 'no idea of the potentially deadly consequences of developing anorexia nervosa' (Bloomfield in Catan & Bennett, 2007) and that 'the site owners don't mention (probably because they don't know themselves) the risk of osteoporosis, the effect on fertility and the hugely increased risk of heart disease or heart failure' (Bloomfield, 2006). Such narratives rest on, once again, an erroneous binary construction. This assumes that pro-anorexia *must* constitute a denial of illness because illness *cannot* incite desire; if they knew the dangers – the realities – participants simply *could not* want anorexia. Viewing pro-anorexia, thus, as underpinned by 'choice', such media coverage resonates with a neoliberal paradigm of responsible citizens; to be rational and responsible, participants to these sites simply 'cannot' know what they are doing. However, this is not supported by participant observation on the sites. Instead, in line with more recent press coverage (cf. Gregoire, September 2012), and as the prevalent trope of support suggests, participants 'know of the dangerous consequences associated with their behaviours but this does not deter them from continuing' (Williams & Reid, 2007: 150). Many pro-anorexia websites contain detailed warnings of anorexia's dangers and inform participants how to identify particular bodily symptoms which suggest that their illness 'has gone too far'. Similarly, there is advice on how to stay alive and maintain a certain level of health *with(in)* – crucially not without – anorexia. This consists of information regarding vitamins and heart health for example. As such, as one website creator put it during fieldwork, pro-anorexia is about 'accepting the side effects but attempting to simply stay alive'. This bleak binary offers a glimpse at the ambivalence that pervades these websites, which draws into question neoliberal notions of 'choice' emphasized by media coverage.

In her interview, Josie wrote: 'I have lost quite a few friends to eating disorders and I live with the physical consequences of anorexia and personally believe that pro ana sites should be made illegal because then at least fewer people would be motivated even more to continue an eating disordered pattern'. And yet, at the time of her interview, Josie was a frequent visitor to the websites and wrote passionately about how she would be 'lost' and 'alone' without them. Josie's ambivalence towards the sites ensues from, and mirrors, that towards the illness itself which was expressed by many informants. In their interviews, as on the websites, articulations of pain and distress shared space with pride at anorexia and a desire to maintain it. Even outright hatred of anorexia does not preclude pro-anorexic desire in informants' narratives; the former may even, paradoxically, underpin the latter, which was illuminated by my interview on the eating disorders unit with Lois. Describing why she strived to maintain anorexia, she said: 'well, I have to be good at something'; and that something, to Lois, was anorexia. This sentiment of adapting to a *lack of* choice by being 'good at' the illness you have is echoed across pro-anorexia websites. Participation in these therefore emerges as being about living – 'making do' (de Certeau, 1984) – with existing illness rather than being a clear-cut expression of choice or 'lifestyle' preference. Materializing here is a key point that has resonated throughout the ethnographic data so far: pro-anorexia websites are not underpinned by the desire to *get* an illness, or even to *get better at* it. They are, rather, all about living through, and holding onto, one's existing diagnosed anorexia.

Many pro-anorexia websites have information sections outlining clinical nosologies of anorexia, bulimia and EDNOS. These comprise listings, usually derived from the DSM IV (APA, 1994), of diagnostic criteria for each. They are accompanied by 'what to expect' paragraphs, which discuss the physical and mental symptoms that 'fulfil' these criteria. In their interviews, some informants recounted a daily practice of (re-)comparing their somatic selves to these criteria to check they were 'still anorexic'. It has been suggested that 'classifications' such as medical diagnoses 'change the ways in which individuals experience themselves' (Hacking, 1999: 104; see also Rose, 2007). However, the temporality within these discussions varies from engagements with diagnostic categories on pro-anorexia websites; the latter are affirmative, not generative. Diagnosis – at its first bestowal as well as at every processual moment of checking thereafter – offers a space to be, as one informant put it, 'stereotypically anorexic'. Through it, personhood and anorexia (re-)merge in ways that are felt to be already subjectively present and yet which become 'legitimately' clinical. The pervasive discourse of authenticity – or, of what we might call 'authenticity-through-biomedicine' – in these engagements demonstrates that pro-anorexia websites are 'biosocialities' (Rabinow, 1999) formed around *existing*, clinically-diagnosed, anorexia, with all the messiness and ambivalence that carries with it. As such, informants' accounts illuminate a disparity between the temporality attributed to these sites by the media and by participants themselves. Whilst the former frame them as spaces of teleological competition to become ever-thinner, the latter describe them instead as allowing participants to live through, and maintain, an existing illness. This latter stance is encapsulated visually by the E.D. ribbon icon that was present on many of the early pro-anorexia websites, and which still remains on some. As well as standing for eating disorders, the ribbon's initials also signified 'end discrimination', and the symbol originated on a website whose name included a reference to healing. As such, these ribbons spoke of an attempt to live with, and through, illness without stigma or judgement as much as of a glorification of ever-increasing anorexia. Like this symbol, participants' narratives do not evince a current lack but, rather, a sense of stasis. To many, pro-anorexia websites are spaces in which they can be alone with illness, unhindered and un-judged, and in which healing may take place *within* ambivalently intransigent anorexia, rather than necessarily signifying a recovery from the illness. Taking account of this temporality of existing anorexia is therefore crucial to any consideration of the sites. Helping participants hold onto and even be 'good at' an illness that many described as a friend (see Lavis, 2013) whilst also knowing how much it damaged them, emerged as the central reason for being on the sites. This shifts how we read features of pro-anorexia websites that are often framed by the media as producing inter-subjective competition.

In her interview, Nancy said of the pro-anorexia website in which she participated:

> It's not a place where others encourage one to be sick, it's a place where one can talk about their woes and what they ate in knowing there's others who are in the same place. In another words, we're really talking to ourselves with an echo of "oh gawd, I did the same".

Although here 'talking to oneself' resonates with the support explored above, in other informants' accounts it elucidated how competition works on the sites, showing it to be intra- not inter-subjective. In her interview, Laura said:

> The pro ana sites help to encourage me to be a "good" anorexic because they often give tips on how to avoid social meal situations and also give tricks on how to hide food etc. if you cannot avoid meals.

Here *Tips & Tricks* do not emerge as modalities of 'turning' others anorexic or, indeed, of making individuals who already have the illness more anorexic, as the media has emphasized. Rather, against the background of participating in the sites to hold onto existing illness as a way of living with it and being 'good at something', *Tips & Tricks* can be seen as ways to negotiate the day-to-day realities of needing food without losing anorexia by eating 'too much'. As such, this is an intra-subjective competition against one's own hunger to maintain and 'live up to' diagnosis. This was also clear when Kyra recounted how every time she visited a new pro-anorexia website she searched for biographical information about the website's creator to check how much they ate and weighed. She described feeling: 'Like I needed to be able to "compete" with them'. Whilst Kyra's words highlight how competition is within the space of one's own anorexia, they also begin to hint at the way in which thinness enters this dynamic of intra-subjective competition in ways more nuanced than the media might imagine.

In informants' accounts, thinness emerges as a marker of anorexia's continuing presence (see Lavis, 2014) rather than as a goal of self-starvation. Many described measuring the size of wrists or thighs, checking today's bodily emaciation against yesterday's, in order to see whether anorexia was 'still present'. Measuring their thinness – both against themselves and others – constitutes a way for individuals to check that, with the help of *Tips & Tricks* perhaps, they have 'successfully' held onto anorexia and still fit the diagnostic criteria. As such, bodily thinness *comes* to be important *within*, or *after*, lived experiences of diagnosed anorexia rather than being an aim of the self-starvation in anorexia. But, it is here, along the body's corporeal perimeters and their visual representation in the form of *Thinspiration* that one of the central encounters between media imaginings and pro-anorexia websites takes place. Having explored prevalent media portrayals of the sites as well as listened to participants' voices, we can now turn to trace the threads of echolalia, engagement, and enactment woven through this encounter. In so doing, the final part of the chapter shows how media representations of anorexia-as-thinness become 'lines of flight' (Deleuze & Guattari, 2004) inscribed with a desire that problematizes participants' own conceptualizations of pro-anorexia and even undermines their lived experiences of the illness itself.

Thinspiration and Misrepresentation*:* A Cyber-landscape Alters

In their interviews, many informants discussed *Thinspiration*, a widespread feature of pro-anorexia websites. Although, at first glance, *Thinspiration* pages may appear to comprise photographs of, simply put, 'thin people', a closer look tells a more complex story that resonates with participants' sense of already-compromised conditions of possibility and the liminal position of thinness in their narratives. Describing her viewing of such images, Nora suggested that 'thinspirational pictures of actual anorexics play a big role in these sites'. Nora's words are crucial to an understanding of *Thinspiration*'s significance both to pro-anorexia websites and to the day-to-day lives of their participants. On these sites 'pictures of actual anorexics' take two forms; the first is in images labelled *Diagnosed Anorexics* or sometimes, *Admitted Anorexics.* These depict celebrities who have 'come out' as anorexic, usually by going into treatment, and are often divided into before and after shots. Yet, unlike in advertisements for plastic surgery or diet products, celebrity *diagnosed anorexics* are lauded for looking the same at these two time points. Their corporeal consistency in visual thinness is, as noted above in relation to my informants, a marker of continuing anorexia. About this genre of *Thinspiration*, Kyra wrote:

> I looked for not just slim models, but bony ones, ones that look ill! Like the size zero and even more for more double zero actresses. Like when Nicole Ritchie and Lindsay Lohan were really skinny and Portia de Rossi was pictured on some red carpet and from behind you could see her ribs.

Kyra's predilection for images of individuals 'that look ill' is important; in line with the discourse of authenticity around diagnosis, it is a legitimately *anorexic* thinness that is key to making these photographs *Thinspirational.* As Nora put it in her interview, 'if I know that the person that I'm looking at is anorexic then it appeals to my competitive side and encourages me to starve myself'. This emphasis on the 'authentic' visuality of anorexia is also found in the second sub-genre of *Thinspiration*, which comprises photographs of participants themselves. In her interview, Laura wrote:

> I think it's important to have pictures of emaciated people and not just thin people because it's a reminder of what I am aspiring to be ... I don't want to

> be thin I want to be emaciated and often the only place to find anorexic looking pictures is on these pro ana sites.

As Laura's words suggest, the recognition that pro-anorexia websites are spaces in which participants can 'be', and work at being, diagnosed anorexics is central to how a specific 'ill' thinness of *Thinspiration* enters subjectivities of desire. Thinness is aspirational – and I argue, *only aspirational* – when it delineates this 'authentic' pathology-identity; as Kyra put it, 'pro-anorexia is the desire to remain *eating disorder thin*' (italics mine). This desire, therefore, is focused on the process of holding onto one's existing eating disorder where that presence is *measured* through thinness; it does not have generic 'weight loss' as a goal.

However, as noted in Part One, *Thinspiration* has been ubiquitous in media coverage of pro-anorexia websites. Emptying these images of their inflections of stasis and pathology-identity, the media has tended to focus on the viewing of 'celebrity bodies' as inspiring weight loss. Assuming that website participants desire to mimetically 'sculpt' their own bodies, the media have suggested that 'pro-anorexic sites have often held up certain celebrities as examples of "thinspiration"' (Howard, 2007: 15). Such coverage positions *Thinspiration* as nothing more than 'photographs of slim (or, indeed, skinny) celebrities and models to serve as motivation for young anorexics to starve themselves' (Closer, unattributed, 2009; see also Burton, 2012; Goodchild, 2006; Nicholl, 2011). This interpretation of *Thinspiration* as centrally *about* thinness and of pro-anorexia website participants as a 'body-obsessed audience' (*Daily Mail*, unattributed, March 21, 2012) can be traced back to very early media coverage, which described 'photos of waifish models and actresses' (Dolan, 2003) and 'pictures of excessively thin people' (BBC, unattributed, 2001) that 'glamorise thinness' (ibid.). As such, it arguably shaped public imaginings of pro-anorexia websites early on in their history and this conceptualization has continued to solidify over time.

Thus, website participants and the media read *Thinspiration*'s images in very different ways. That these are seen by the latter as contagious – illustrated by discussions of 'predators' explored above – and also as one-dimensionally about thinness offers insights into media imaginings not only of pro-anorexia websites but also of anorexia nervosa. To claim, for example, that 'Victoria Beckham is revered as a "thinspiration" by women with anorexia' (Wilson, E., 2006) entangles both anorexia and the websites into wider discussions of weight loss and, specifically, of size zero (see Atkins, 2002; Howard, 2007; Spencer, 2006; Wilson, E., 2006). This was sometimes pointed out by informants themselves; in her interview, Miriam, an inpatient in the eating disorders unit, said with frustration:

> There's lots of people who think it's just a vanity thing like, you know, anorexia is just the thinness and wanting to look thin but it's not a vanity thing, it's not at all. People go "oh everyone's trying to copy this size zero trend" and it's not, it's not! You don't open a picture … look at a picture, and say "oh I must look like

> that girl, therefore I must lose weight, therefore I'm an anorexic!" It's absolutely nothing to do with that.

The merging together of subjectively and temporally different thinnesses in such media discussions blurs any felt and lived distinction between anorexia and dieting. It overlooks the centrality of a relationship between what is seen and what is felt when website participants engage with *Thinspiration*. It thereby flattens and ignores the specific desirability of 'anorexic emaciation' as a marker of legitimate anorexia, and the ways in which this comes to be important through the conditions of possibility set out by existing illness. As such, media coverage resonates with what Jodie Allen has termed the pervasive cultural 'spectacularization of the anorexic subject position' (2008). Allen argues that certain media portrayals of anorexia posit an 'end-stage' and 'ahistorical' body as 'the *ultimate* signification of *the* anorexic subject position' (Allen, 2008: 589, italics in original). This, she suggests, incites desire in individuals with anorexia for the subject-position embodied in this end-stage body. In relation to pro-anorexia websites, this is both true and yet not. Certainly media discussions of *Thinspiration* do engender desire but, importantly, *not* in individuals already living through anorexia. Rather, they make pro-anorexia desirable from what we might term 'outside anorexia' by advertising the illness as a means-to-an-end teleological 'weight loss' tool and pro-anorexia websites as the places to 'go and catch it'. This is rendered more powerful by the fact that it is still not uncommon for media discussions to cite the names of the websites themselves (cf. Gotthelf, 2001; Robinson, 2012).

In her interview, Laura demonstrated the advertising potential of media coverage when she said: 'I have always known that pro ana sites existed because I had seen them mentioned in the media'. Putting Laura's words in context for us, Aurelie, whom we met at the beginning of the chapter, wrote:

> Why there are ever expanding members since it started? If you look back, the newspapers/TV talk shows/news/magazines merely glorified it. Nowadays, it seems like it is being seen as a fad. If you want to be cool and lose weight fast, be anorexic. And given the huge media attention, all these youngsters these days will simply google them up.

The 'youngsters' Aurelie describes are commonly called *wannarexics*, both on pro-anorexia websites and in the media. As Boero and Pascoe have recently written, 'the wannarexic treats anorexia as a fad, something that can be adopted and discarded at will' (2012: 39). It was about these new visitors to the websites that AnaGirlEmpath, a pro-anorexia blogger and researcher, who kindly shared her thoughts with me in online conversations in 2012–13, wrote:

> The Wanarexia Phenomenon is the unfortunate self-fulfilled prophecy of Mass Media. Wanarexics were scarcely seen before the first wave of serious condemnation in 2001. Before this, ProAna had an inconspicuous presence

> online; only those who already had ED's were likely to come across ProAna content. After awareness and condemnation of the Movement was presented to the masses, we began to see a vast influx of individuals who did NOT have ED's but either 1) coveted ED's because of an impression that ED's are "cool" or "fashionable", and therefore literally, actively trying to create an ED in themselves; and 2) people hoping to garner "tips and tricks" to lose weight.

After being visited by *wannarexics* during fieldwork in 2012, the homepage of one pro-anorexia website read: 'we have seen a disturbing influx of individuals drawn to [our site] for the wrong reasons and a distortion in the general conceptualization of what ProAna is all about'. The use of the word 'distortion' here is interesting, and key to an understanding of how the media have actively and concretely altered the landscape of pro-anorexia websites.

Wannarexics not only transiently visit these websites to ask how to be anorexic and lose weight. Rather, just like existing participants, these new visitors also 'hang around' and they do so in ways not always so silent. In fact, participant observation on the sites demonstrated that *wannarexics* both initiate and join conversations as well as upload and exchange what they regard as *thinspirational* images. These latter alter the character of *Thinspiration* pages, exchanging a focus on legitimately anorexic emaciation for one on weight loss. As far back as 2004, *Ana's Girls*, a book describing itself as *The Essential Guide to the Underground Eating Disorders Community Online*, charted this emergence of two types of *Thinspiration* with completely opposing meanings; it suggested: 'Thinspiration may be more or less graphic. Groups that aim for emaciation will be more likely to display photographs of women suffering from malnutrition whereas groups that aim for a more mainstream ideal of beauty will post photographs of celebrities such as Britney Spears' (Uca, 2004: 14). As more content becomes focused on celebrities' thinness, the temporality and emphases of pro-anorexia websites alter; ways to become thin replace those to 'make do' (de Certeau, 1984) with existing illness. In contrast to the 'storied sociality' (Stewart, 1996), described above, the sites' multi-dimensionality, complexity and ambivalence flatten into a quest for size zero and thigh gaps. As such, it is *after* the media and from *outside* anorexia that it begins to *become* true that on pro-anorexia websites 'there is often extreme or dangerous dieting advice given which promote harmful behaviours' (Bond, 2012: 2). Moreover, as the media report on this new differently-shaped teleological 'pro-anorexia' as *the* pro-anorexia, more *wannarexics* flock to the sites and this 'new pro-anorexia' solidifies into 'fact'. Writing about *wannarexics,* Aurelie argued: 'a lot of folks in these groups are really teeny boppers, teens, young adults who don't know what they're getting into'. In her emphasis on the unknowingness, age and gender of participants, as in her use of the verb 'glorify' above, we see that in this media-generated process of change, both the participants to, and contents of, pro-anorexia websites become what the media always claimed them to be. As such, in the relationship between pro-anorexia websites and the media, 'it is the map that engenders the territory' (Baudrillard, 1983: 2). Furthermore, as the lived, contextual and ambivalent pro-anorexia of website participants is overlaid in this way, the word 'pro-anorexia' is reconfigured and repopulated not only on these websites, but across the landscape of cyberspace.

Just before *Pinterest* banned content it regarded as pro-anorexic in 2012, *The Daily Mail* drew attention to such content by arguing that individuals 'who post pictures of emaciated women as a way to encourage fellow die-hard dieters' (*Daily Mail*, unattributed, March 21, 2012) had infiltrated *Pinterest*, which it described as 'another fertile breeding ground for pro-anorexia' (ibid.). Likewise, a spokesperson from B-eat (formerly the UK's Eating Disorders Association) told *The Telegraph* in 2013 that 'it's worrying that with the powerful medium of social networking and the growing popularity of phone apps such as *Instagram*, people are able to easily access images that encourage the individual to believe that an eating disorder is a lifestyle choice and to avoid treatment' (Philipson, 2013; see also Styles, 2013). Although illustrating, once again, the ways in which the media pervasively blur a desire for weight loss with anorexia, these reports also tell a further story. Here, they not only (re-)produce this textually through their own reporting, but also document the blurring as it takes place across cyberspace. Thus when a headline reads, 'those caught up in thigh gap obsession have plenty of fuel for their mania', and the article describes how *Tumblr*, *Twitter* and *Facebook* all have 'pages devoted to posting images' (Miller, 2013), and it terms these 'pro-anorexic', they are – of sorts. This 'new pro-anorexia', thus, spills across the web, coming to life in other spaces and forms of media, taking on increasing solidity in each incarnation. This seepage is also not limited only to online worlds; a search for 'pro ana' or 'pro-anorexia' on Amazon.co.uk uncovers texts such as *All things thin and beautiful: Discover a whole new meaning to pro ana* (Martin, 2012) and *Beauty is slim and lean: Living PRO ANA the healthy way* (Charles, 2013). The ways in which such spaces and texts utilize this new form of 'pro-anorexia' suggest, moreover, that as a new pro-anorexia is defined and brought to life across these diverse forms of media, so too is a 'new anorexia'.

I argued above that media interpretations of *Thinspiration* as about nothing more than the quest for bodily thinness simplistically elided anorexia with a wider cultural obsession with dieting and weight loss. Now emerging from, and held up by, this cyber-landscape that claims pro-anorexia as its own is a simulacrous, 'spectacular' and 'hyperreal' (Baudrillard, 1983) anorexia – one that is indeed focused on dieting and weight loss and which privileges the visual over the subjective. Like the dislocated, emptied 'new pro-anorexia' that frames and invigorates it, this is a de-relational anorexia of surface, invested with, and related to, nothing but bodily thinness. It is, to borrow from Deleuze, 'a hecceity [...] as opposed to a subjectivity' (Deleuze, 2007: 130) and one, moreover, that clashes both with informants' lived experiences and with clinical realities and categories. With the 'hecceity' comes a subject position desired and inhabited by *wannarexics* but refuted by pro-anorexia website participants themselves who risk being left out – abjected even – by its pervasive online presence. Thus, *wannarexics*, and the new media-generated pro-anorexia and anorexia that come increasingly to life around them, are argued by pro-anorexia website participants both to threaten their 'identity and well-being', as David Giles (2006: 472) has highlighted, and to harmfully (re-)shape public perceptions of eating disorders. The *wannarexic*-desired 'new anorexia' is felt to undermine the status of anorexia nervosa as legitimate illness, thereby ignoring the suffering and lack of choice that accompanies individuals' lived experiences of it. Thus, although pro-anorexia website participants find themselves unable to control either the media or the imaginings of anorexia and pro-anorexia that the media engender and circulate in 'public culture' (Ortner, 2006), they do attempt to keep these out of pro-anorexia websites, thereby limiting the extent to which they may vie for space with participants' own eating disorders. In a conjoined patrolling of clinical and cyber boundaries thus, and in contrast to press imaginings of 'predators' turning 'victims' anorexic, there has been a frustrated and hostile response to *wannarexics*.

In our online discussions during fieldwork, AnaGirlEmpath, whom we met above, suggested that:

> Many Admins of ProAna Communities have taken a proactive stance against the accessibility of wanarexics to our Communities. Contrary to popular (media-propagated) misconception, ED sufferers do NOT want to recruit ANYONE to the path of pathology. The Wanarexic Phenomenon is highly disturbing and offensive to most ED sufferers, and many communities go out of their way to deter such individuals from staying.

As AnaGirlEmpath's words suggest, visitors to the sites asking how to become anorexic in order to lose weight are widely discouraged; the tagline to one site reads: 'do not visit our site or forum if you are hoping to develop an eating disorder or wish to lose a few pounds. We believe that an eating disorder does NOT constitute a lifestyle choice, but a terrible and life threatening disease'. As this quotation elucidates, discouragement often highlights the horror and pain of anorexia, accentuating the very aspects of the illness on which the websites' key trope of support centres. And, just as those discussions mingled pain, pride and a sense of authenticity, it is this triangulation that reappears here. In opposition to *wannarexics*, participants emphasize their own subjectivities of having 'always been anorexic' and having 'no choice'. In her interview, Aurelie said: 'in the Pro-Anorexia groups these days, mainly it's all about learning HOW to have an eating disorder. What they don't understand is that you can't GET an eating disorder'. Both the clinical legitimacy and equally real suffering of diagnosed anorexia, which we saw earlier, here become a modality of boundary patrolling. They denote *wannarexics* as 'other' – unwelcome and 'inauthentic'. As one informant in the eating disorders unit who was also a pro-anorexia website participant, Elle, put it in a discussions of *wannarexics*: 'If you're anorexic, then you do not need tips on how to not eat'. Authenticity through diagnosis is thus discursively re-solidified and (re)inhabited against 'outsiders'.

It might have been noticed that the tense of this discussion has been in the present both 'before' and 'after' the media-generated alterations to the landscape of pro-anorexia websites and the anorexia(s) that vie for space in this ever-shifting terrain. Such linguistic mingling ensues from, and draws attention to, the fact that such changes are not one moment events. They are, rather, continual processes that have been absorbed into the dynamics of these websites, causing their participants to continually react against them. Yet, alongside the boundary patrolling of existing pro-anorexia sites, there has also been a more permanent alteration to their landscape, which does require some differentiation between tenses. The threats felt by participants to be posed by the media-generated visitors to the sites have rendered spaces of stasis paradoxically mobile; like the evacuation of a ruined landscape, many informants describe having abandoned the websites and instead joined or formed new ones. In order to distinguish these websites from the spaces of spectacular anorexia and the teleological 'new pro-anorexia', as well as to keep them hidden from *wannarexics*, many are increasingly labelled pro-acceptance rather than pro-anorexia. As Aurelie put it in her interview:

> Many older and wiser members were tired of the bombarded messages of "Help, I need to lose 10 lbs in a week" and think that if they just eat apples for a week ... voila they're anorexic!!! (note the sarcastic tone) So, those folks (I'm one of them) decided to form our own forums. We coined the term "Pro-Acceptance", because there were all sorts of folks who are in various stages of their disorder. In these types of groups, they are either still ravaged by this disease, in a place where they are "living" with the disease, or in recovery.

Describing itself as having been a pro-anorexia website but now terming itself 'pro-acceptance', one homepage advises its participants that it 'strive[s] to offer love and support to all our members in whatever they are going through in their lives. The only proviso is that to join the forum you must be suffering from an eating disorder and over 15 years of age'. The advent of pro-acceptance thus utilizes diagnostic classification to maintain the presence of spaces in which those living through anorexia and other eating disorders can be alone with their illnesses in the wider context of 'storied sociality' (Stewart, 1996). However, this move towards pro-acceptance also enables pro-anorexia websites to continue to more permanently transform into the media template held up for them; they (have) become 'alarming' spaces revolving around the production of thin bodies. This leaves very particular, and potentially harmful, imaginings of both pro-anorexia and anorexia intact and continuing to circulate in 'public culture' (Ortner, 2006).

Conclusion: Alarm and the Doubling of Abjection

By exploring pro-anorexia websites through ethnography and interviews with participants to the sites, this chapter has engaged with the complexities and ambivalence that underpin these spaces. Accounts of 'hanging out' in cyberspace have drawn our attention to the ways in which being pro-anorexic may be about living through illness and reconfiguring already severely compromised conditions of possibility; it is a desire to maintain one's illness and be 'good at something' that instigates the sites' dynamics of intra-subjective competition. Such narratives pose a challenge to media imaginings of pro-anorexia websites as populated by 'victims' and 'predators' caught up in the constantly-mobile pursuit of ever-increasing anorexia. The chapter traced how underscoring this illusory binary is a conceptualization of both pro-anorexia websites and anorexia itself as centrally *about* thinness. By viewing this illness simply as a teleological and contagious quest for emaciated limbs and thigh gaps, the media positions the websites as spaces both formed around, and in which to 'catch', extreme weight-loss. Yet, as this chapter has suggested, such media imaginings are not only documentary but also performative; tracing alterations to the landscape of these websites has illuminated the (re-)shaping, reification and cultural leakage of a 'new pro-anorexia' and has shown how its accompanying 'new anorexia' becomes invigorated and invested with desire by the media's words. As such, within patrolled bodily perimeters, as well as across the diverse locations in which this 'new pro-anorexia' manifests, simulated and dissimulated, diagnosed and discursive, spectral and lived, anorexias all vie for space and both clinical and cultural legitimacy. As this constructed and spectacular 'new anorexia' is sought after and inhabited by *wannarexics*, both the clinical legitimacy of eating disorders and the importance of this to individuals who are living through and holding onto these illnesses, are threatened. Importantly, in addition to problematizing any straightforward singular conceptualization of 'pro-anorexia' these media-generated processes can be seen to instigate a concomitant dynamic of abjection. Endangering sanctuary spaces, albeit those mingling support with 'negative enabling' (Haas et al., 2011), and problematizing individuals' lived anorexia both serve to displace participants, setting them apart from their illness and themselves; they are offered no place 'to be' either in cyberspace or 'public culture' (Ortner, 2006). As such, these processes arguably double the already-present abjection and entrapment ensuing from the illness itself, which participants' engagements with the 'storied sociality' (Stewart, 1996) of pro-anorexia websites were attempts to mediate. Thus, whilst pro-anorexia is a phenomenon boosted, produced, tangled and obscured by every word written about it, such textual performances potentially also leave individuals with eating disorders more in need of support and increasingly hidden, as well as both doubly-abject and profoundly mired in cultural alarm.

Acknowledgements

The PhD research on which this chapter draws was undertaken in the Anthropology Department at Goldsmiths, University of London and I thank my supervisors there, Dr Simon Cohn and Professor Catherine Alexander. The PhD was funded by an

Economic and Social Research Council studentship and a Goldsmiths Bursary. It won the 2010 Radcliffe-Brown/Sutasoma Award from the Royal Anthropological Institute. I should like to express my gratitude to the many individuals who have shared their stories about, and views of, pro-anorexia websites with me, and to thank AnaGirlEmpath for our research discussions about pro-anorexia.

References

Allen, J.T. (2008). The spectacularization of the anorexic subject position. *Current Sociology*, *56*, 587–603.

APA (1994). *Diagnostic and statistical manual of mental disorders IV.* Washington, DC: American Psychiatric Association.

Asthana, A. (2007, January 7). 'Danger of the websites that promote anorexia'. *The Observer* [online]. Retrieved from http://www.guardian.co.uk/technology/2007/jan/07/news.medicineandhealth [accessed April 8, 2013].

Atkins, L. (2002, July 23). 'It's better to be thin and dead than fat and living'. *The Guardian* [online]. Retrieved from http://www.guardian.co.uk/print/0,4466711-103409,00.html [accessed April 8, 2013].

Back, L. (2007). *The art of listening.* Oxford & New York: Berg.

Bardone-Cone, A. & Cass, K. (2006). Investigating the impact of pro-anorexia websites: A pilot study. *European Eating Disorders Review*, *14*, 256–262.

Barnett, E. (2012, August 3). Pinterest tackles eating disorders. *The Daily Telegraph* [online]. Retrieved from http://www.telegraph.co.uk/technology/socialmedia/9449049/Pinterest-tackles-eating-disorders.html [accessed January 20, 2013].

Barnett, E. (2012, October 15). Does the internet encourage eating disorders? *The Daily Telegraph* [online]. Retrieved from http://www.telegraph.co.uk/women/womens-life/9609534/Does-the-internet-encourage-eating-disorders.html [accessed January 20, 2013].

Baudrillard, J. (1983). *Simulations*. New York: Semiotext(e).

BBC, unattributed (2001, May 24). 'Anorexia websites "glamorise thinness"'. *BBC News* [online]. Retrieved from http://news.bbc.co.uk/2/hi/health/1348665.stm [accessed April 8, 2013].

BBC, unattributed (2005, February 8). 'BBC Probe into Anorexia Websites'. *BBC News* [online]. Retrieved from http://news.bbc.co.uk/l/hi/wales/425109.stm [accessed July 26, 2011].

BBC, unattributed (2007, January 6). 'Warning over pro-anorexia sites'. *BBC News* [online]. Retrieved from http://news.bbc.co.uk/l/hi/uk/6236529.stm [accessed May 18, 2011].

Bell, M. (2009). '@ the doctor's office': Pro-anorexia and the medical gaze. *Surveillance & Society*, *6*, 151–162.

Black, A. (2012). *How to be anorexic: A pro-ana handbook.* Kindle ebook.

Bloomfield, S. (2006). *Pro anna websites: Press release.* London: The Eating Disorders Association.

Boero, N. & Pascale, C.J. (2012). Pro-anorexia communities and online interaction: Bringing the pro-ana body online. *Body & Society*, *18*, 27–57.

Bond, E. (2012, November 28). *Virtually anorexic – where's the harm? A research study on the risks of pro-anorexia websites*. London: B-eat, Childnet International, Nominet Trust.

Borzekowski, D.L.G., Schenk, S., Wilson, J.L. & Peebles, R. (2010). E-Ana and e-Mia: A content analysis of pro-eating disorder websites. *American Journal of Public Health*, *100*, 1526–1534.

Boycott, R. (2008). Investigation: The truth about anorexia websites that helped drive a 13-year-old to suicide. *The Daily Mail* [online]. Retrieved from http://www.dailymail.co.uk/femail/article-1089765/Investigation-The-truth-anorexia-websites-helped-drive-13-year-old-suicide.html [accessed January 10, 2013].

Bray, A. (1996). The anorexic body: Reading disorders. *Cultural Studies*, *10*, 413–429.

Brown, J. (2001, July 23). '"The winner dies": A web-based pro-anorexia movement provides a bizarre support network for starving girls'. *The Salon* [online]. Retrieved from http://www.salon.com/2001/07/23/pro_ana/ [accessed April 8, 2013].

Burke, E. (2009). Pro-anorexia and the Internet: A tangled web of representation and (dis)embodiment. *Counselling, Psychotherapy, and Health*, *5*, 60–81.

Burton, I. (2012, November 30). The pro-anorexia sites that offer deadly 'thinspiration'. *The Independent* [online]. Retrieved from http://www.independent.co.uk/voices/comment/the-proanorexia-sites-that-offer-deadly-thinspiration-8371885.html [accessed January 21, 2013].

Catan, T. & Bennett, R. (2007, January 8). 'Spain takes lead in closing down the websites that tell girls it's good to be an anorexic'. *The Times* [online]. Retrieved from http://www.timesonline.co.uk/article/0,8122-2536634.html [accessed July 27, 2011].

Charles, A. (2013). *Beauty is slim and lean: Living PRO ANA the healthy way.* Kindle E-Book.

Closer, unattributed (2009, April 9). Fearne's anorexia shocker. *Closer Magazine* [online]. Retrieved from http://www.closeronline.co.uk/ShowbizNews/LatestNews/fearne-cottons-anorexia-shocker.aspx [accessed January 20, 2013].

Courtney-Smith, N. (2006, June 29). The cult of anorexia. *The Daily Mail.* Retrieved from http://www.mailonsunday.co.uk/pages/live/femail/article.html?in_article_id=393037&in_page_id=1879 [accessed May 4, 2011].

Daily Mail, unattributed (2007, January 6). 'Pro-anorexia websites killing people'. *The Daily Mail* [online]. Retrieved from http://www.dailymail.co.uk/news/article-426836/Pro-anorexia-websites-killing-people.html [accessed January 20, 2013].

Daily Mail, unattributed (2012, March 21). '"The site lends itself remarkably well to thinspiration boards": Pinterest under pressure to crack down on pro-anorexia use'. *The Daily Mail* [online]. Retrieved from http://www.dailymail.

co.uk/femail/article-2118256/Pinterest-pressure-crack-pro-anorexia-use.html [accessed April 10, 2013].

Daily Mail, unattributed (2012, March 26). Pinterest bans pro-anorexia content after pressure to crack down on 'thinspiration' boards. *The Daily Mail* [online]. Retrieved from http://www.dailymail.co.uk/femail/article-2120634/Pinterest-bans-pro-anorexia-content-pressure-crack-thinspiration-boards.html [accessed January 20, 2013].

Davies, P. & Lipset, Z. (2003). Ana's gone surfing. *The Psychologist*, *16*, 424–425.

De Certeau, M. (1984). *The practice of everyday life.* Berkeley & London: University of California Press.

Deleuze, G. (2007). *Two regimes of madness: Texts and interview 1975–1995.* New York: Semiotext(e).

Deleuze, G. & Guattari, F. (2004). *A Thousand Plateaus: Capitalism and Schizophrenia.* London & New York: Continuum.

Dias, K. (2003). The ana sanctuary: Women's pro-anorexia narratives in cyberspace. *Journal of International Women's Studies*, *4*, 31–45.

Dolan, D. (2003, February 2). 'Learning to love anorexia? "Pro ana" websites flourish'. *The New York Observer* [online]. Retrieved from http://observer.com/2003/02/learning-to-love-anorexia-proana-web-sites-flourish/ [accessed April 9, 2013].

Doward, J. & Reilly, T. (2003, August 17). 'How macabre world of the web offers fresh insight on anorexics'. *The Observer* [online]. Retrieved from http://www.guardian.co.uk/news/2003/aug/17/medicineandhealth.society [accessed April 8, 2013].

Driscoll, B. (2012, November 29). 'Pro-ana sites encourage extreme dieting and eating disorders in girls'. *Huffington Post* [online]. Retrieved from http://www.huffingtonpost.co.uk/2012/11/29/pro-anorexia-websites-young-girls-eating-disorder_n_2209959.html [accessed January 21, 2013].

Elliott, C. (2004). *Better than well: American medicine meets the American dream.* New York & London: W.W. Norton & Co.

Ellis, A. (2012). *Thinspo: A novel.* CreateSpace Independent Publishing Platform.

Epstein, S. (1996) *Impure science: AIDS, activism, and the politics of knowledge.* Berkeley & London: University of California Press.

Evans, J. (2011). *Becoming John: Anorexia's not just for girls.* Bloomington, Indiana: Xlibris Corporation.

Fox, S. (2011). The social life of health information. *Pew internet and American life project* [online]. Retrieved from http://www.pewInternet.org/Reports/2011/Social-Life-of-Health-Info/Summary-of-Findings.aspx [accessed April 2, 2013].

Gibbon, S. & Novas, C. (eds) (2008). *Biosocialities, genetics and the social sciences: Making biologies and identities.* London & New York: Routledge.

Giles, D. (2006). Constructing identities in cyberspace: The case of eating disorders. *British Journal of Social Psychology*, *45*, 463–477.

Girtz, B. (2013, January 9). 'New report reveals real dangers of "pro-ana" websites'. *Technocrati.com.* [online] Retrieved from http://technorati.com/life style/article/new-report-reveals-real-dangers-of/ [accessed January 20, 2013]

Goodchild, S. (2006, October 30). 'How pro-anorexic porn's poisonous diet "thinspires" young women to waste away'. *Independent.i.e.* [online]. Retrieved from http://independent.i.e./opinion/analysis/how-proanorexic-porns-poisono us-diet-thinspires-young-women-to-waste-away-75793.html [accessed July 20, 2011].

Gotthelf, M. (2001, May 7). 'Sick world of pro-anorexia Internet sites'. *New York Post* [online]. Retrieved from http://www.nypost.com/p/news/item_MsInLMVryNjKJAeIMDKmKL/1 [accessed April 8, 2013].

Gregoire, C. (2012, September 2). 'The hunger blogs: A secret world of teenage "Thinspiration"'. *Huffington Post* [online]. Retrieved from http://www.huffingtonpost.com/2012/02/08/thinspiration-blogs_n_1264459.html [accessed January 20, 2013].

Gregoire, C. (2012, October 8). '*Pinterest* removes eating disorder-related content, pro-anorexia community continues to thrive'. *Huffington Post* [online]. Retrieved from http://www.huffingtonpost.com/2012/08/10/pinterest-removes-eating-disorder-content_n_1747279.html [accessed January 20, 2013].

Haas, S., Irr, M., Jennings, N. & Wagner, L. (2011). Communicating thin: A grounded model of Online Negative Enabling Support Groups in the pro-anorexia movement. *New Media & Society*, *13*, 40–57.

Hacking, I. (1999). *The social construction of what?* Cambridge, MA & London: Harvard University Press.

Halse Anderson, L. (2009). *Wintergirls*. New York: Speak, Penguin Books USA.

Howard, B. (2007, March 17–23). 'Louise is the new pin-up for anorexics'. *Reveal Magazine*, 14–15.

Independent, unattributed (2012, November 28). '"Thinspiration"? Concern over spread of pro-anorexia sites'. *The Independent* [online]. Retrieved from http://www.independent.co.uk/hei-fi/entertainment/thinspiration-concern-over-spread-of-proanorexia-sites-8363583.html [accessed January 21, 2013].

Kellener, D. (1994). Self-help groups and their relationship to medicine. In J. Gabe, D. Kellener & G. Wiliams (eds), *Challenging medicine.* London: Routledge.

Laurance, J. (2012, November 28). 'Hundreds of websites urging girls to "starve for perfection"'. *The Independent* [online]. Retrieved from http://www.independent.co.uk/life-style/health-and-families/health-news/hundreds-of-websites-urging-girls-to-starve-for-perfection-8360545.html [accessed January 21, 2013].

Lavis, A. (2013). The substance of absence: Exploring eating and anorexia. In E.-J. Abbots & A. Lavis (eds), *Why we eat, how we eat: Contemporary encounters between foods and bodies* (pp. 35–52). Farnham: Ashgate.

Lavis, A. (2014). Engrossing encounters: Materialities and metaphors of fat in the lived experiences of individuals with anorexia. In C. Forth & A. Leitch (eds), *Fat, culture and materiality.* London: Berg.

Lipinski, K. (2007, June 11). 'I was an Internet anorexic'. *Grazia Magazine*, 60–64.

Manning, S. (2012, October 21). 'Self-harm websites top list of teenagers' greatest worries about the internet'. *The Independent* [online]. Retrieved from http://www.independent.co.uk/life-style/gadgets-and-tech/news/selfharm-websites-top-list-of-teenagers-greatest-worries-about-the-internet-8219597.html [accessed April 4, 2013].

Martin, C. (2012). *All things thin and beautiful: Discover a whole new meaning to pro ana.* Kindle E-Book.

Meredith, L. (2012, August 20). 'Pro-anorexia blogs could lead to recovery'. *Tech News Daily* [online]. Retrieved from http://www.technewsdaily.com/4728-pro-anorexia-blogs-could-lead-to-recovery.html [accessed January 17, 2013].

Miah, A. & Rich, E. (2008). *The medicalization of cyberspace.* Oxford & New York: Routledge.

Mikhaylenko, K. (2012). *Glossed.* Kindle E-Book.

Miller, T. (2013, April 1). '"Thigh gap" among the latest unhealthy fixations for the body-obsessed'. *New York Daily News* [online]. Retrieved from http://www.nydailynews.com/life-style/health/thigh-gap-latest-unhealthy-thinspiration-article-1.1304922 [accessed April 4, 2013].

Morris, B.R. (2002, June 23). 'A disturbing growth industry: Web sites that espouse anorexia'. *The New York Times* [online]. Retrieved from http://www.nytimes.com/2002/06/23/health/a-disturbing-growth-industry-web-sites-that-espouse-anorexia.htmlpro%20ana%20web?pagewanted=2 [accessed April 8, 2013].

Mulveen, R. & Hepworth, J. (2006). An interpretive phenomenological analysis of participation in a pro-anorexia Internet site and its relationship with disordered eating. *Journal of Health Psychology*, *11*, 283–296.

Nicholl, K. (2011, August 21). 'Anger as Kate hailed as pro-anorexia role model on U.S. websites'. *The Daily Mail* [online] Retrieved from http://www.dailymail.co.uk/femail/article-2028358/Kate-Middleton-Anger-pro-anorexia-websites-hail-role-model.html [accessed April 4, 2013]

Ortner, S. (2006). *Anthropology and social theory: Culture, power, and the acting subject.* Durham, NC: Duke University Press.

Philipson, A. (2013, January 3). 'Concerns raised over Instagram after app allows users to see photos promoting anorexia'. *The Telegraph* [online]. Retrieved from http://www.telegraph.co.uk/technology/social-media/9775559/Concerns-raised-over-Instagram-after-app-allows-users-to-see-photos-promoting-anorexia.html [accessed April 4, 2013].

Piotrowski, D. (2013, April 4). 'Pro-anorexia culture "explodes" on Instagram, says charity'. *News.com.au* [online]. Retrieved from http://www.news.com.au/lifestyle/health-fitness/thinstagram-warning-how-app-promotes-anorexia/story-fneuzlbd-1226612597060 [accessed April 4, 2013].

Pollack, D. (2003). Pro-eating disorder websites: What should be the feminist response? *Feminism & Psychology*, *13*, 246–251.

Rabinow, P. (1999). Artificiality and enlightenment: From sociobiology to biosociality. In M. Biagiolo (ed.), *The science studies reader.* New York & London: Routledge.

Reaves, J. (2001, July 31). 'Anorexia goes high tech'. *Time* [online]. Retrieved from http://www.time.com/time/health/article/0,8599,169660,00.html [accessed January 21, 2013].

Robinson, M. (2012, November 28). 'One in five girls who have visited a pro-anorexia (or competitive dieting) website are aged 6–11, researchers reveal'. *Daily Mail* [online]. Retrieved from http://www.dailymail.co.uk/news/article-2239645/Hundreds-pro-anorexia-websites-urging-young-girls-competitive-dieting.html#ixzz2Pt56aDe6 [accessed April 8, 2013].

Rose, N. (2007). *The politics of life itself: Biomedicine, power, and subjectivity in the twenty-first century.* Princeton: Princeton University Press.

Schmidt, U. & Treasure, J. (2006). Anorexia Nervosa: Valued and visible. A cognitive-interpersonal maintenance model and its implications for research and practice. *British Journal of Clinical Psychology, 45*, 343–366.

Sontag, S. (2002). *Illness as metaphor and AIDS and its metaphors.* London: Penguin Classics.

Spencer, M. (2006, August 6). The shape we're in: Why women are to blame for our obsession with being thin. *The Observer* [online]. Retrieved from http://www.guardian.co.uk/lifeandstyle/2006/aug/06/healthandwellbeing.features [accessed April 10, 2013].

Stewart, K. (1996). *A space on the side of the road: Cultural poetics in an 'other' America.* Princeton, New Jersey: Princeton University Press.

Styles, R. (2013). 'Instagram attempts to stamp out hashtags that encourage eating disorders – but campaigners demand more action'. *Daily Mail* [online]. Retrieved from http://www.dailymail.co.uk/femail/article-2257111/Instagram-attempts-stamp-hashtags-encourage-eating-disorders--EVER-stop-disturbing-trend.html#ixzz2IXa0dGaz [accessed January 20, 2013].

Thornicroft, G. (2006). *Shunned: Discrimination against people with mental illness.* Oxford: Oxford University Press.

Townsend, C. (2013, March 14). 'Human meat recipes, asphyxiation fan groups and WOMEN who post self-mutilation pictures: My glimpse inside the terrifying cyber world that captivated NYPD's Cannibal Cop'. *Daily Mail* [online]. Retrieved from http://www.dailymail.co.uk/news/article-2289784/Human-meat-recipes-asphyxiation-fan-groups-WOMEN-post-self-mutilation-pictures-My-glimpse-inside-terrifying-cyber-world-captivated-NYPDs-Cannibal-Cop.html?ito=feeds-newsxml [accessed April 4, 2013].

Uca, E.R. (2004). *Ana's girls: The essential guide to the underground eating disorders community online.* Bloomington, Indiana: Author House.

Udovitch, M. (2002, September 8). 'A secret society of the starving'. *The New York Times* [online]. Retrieved from http://www.nytimes.com/2002/09/22/magazine/l-a-secret-society-of-the-starving-923656.html [accessed April 9, 2013].

Williams, S. & Reid, M. (2007). A grounded theory approach to the phenomenon of pro-Anorexia. *Addiction Research & Theory*, *15*, 141–152.
Wilson, E. (2006, June 29). 'The Lovely Bones'. *The Guardian* [online]. Retrieved from http://www.guardian.co.uk/media/2006/jun/29/lifeandhealth.bigbrother [accessed April 10, 2010].
Wilson, J., Peebles, R., Hardy, K. & Litt, I. (2006). Surfing for thinness: A pilot study of pro-eating disorders web site usage in adolescents with eating disorders. *Pediatrics*, *118*, 1635–1643.
Wostear, S. (2007, August 3). 'Sick anorexia websites'. *The Sun.* [online] Retrieved from http://www.thesun.co.uk/sol/homepage/woman/34581/.html [accessed January 19, 2013].
Yeshua-Katz, D. & Martins, N. (2012). Communicating stigma: The pro-ana paradox. *Health Communication* [Epub ahead of print], 1–10.
Ziebland, S. & Wyke, S. (2012). Health and illness in a connected world: How might sharing experiences on the Internet affect people's health? *The Millbank Quarterly*, *90*, 219–249.

Chapter 3
Obesity in the US Media, 1990–2011: Broad Strokes, Broad Consequences

Natalie C. Boero

Introduction

In the United States, the media attention given to obesity is unprecedented, constant and central to the construction of obesity as one of the greatest social problems facing the nation and the world in the twenty-first century. For more than 20 years, the mainstream media in the US have been reporting that obesity and overweight have reached epidemic proportions. Almost daily, obesity and its purported costs and consequences are featured prominently in US media. Even a cursory look through US newspapers clearly shows that the media's obsession with all things obesity-related shows little sign of slowing.

Many social scientists have reported on how media over-reporting on phenomena such as violent crime, child abduction, teenage pregnancy and road rage has created a 'culture of fear', that, in turn, contributes to ever-increasing media coverage of these issues to the effect that problems like poverty go under reported (Cohen, 1972; Glassner, 2000; Boero, 2012). Obesity is no exception; indeed, it is perhaps the best example of the tenacity of this type of over-reporting as the supposed epidemic crossed the 20-year mark with no abatement in coverage in sight. Others have applied this observation to the US media's focus on obesity in an era of growing economic and social inequality, pointing to how an individualized focus on weight takes the focus off of social determinants of health, particularly race and class. The media are also central to the development of obesity as a 'moral panic',[1] as the claims of moral entrepreneurs are publicized and spread through the media to the effect that obesity comes to be seen as a widespread social threat, and overweight and obese people become targets not only of social discrimination and scorn but also of punitive social policy (Goode & Ben-Yehuda, 1994; Boero, 2012).

1 A moral panic occurs when a phenomenon, occurrence, individual, or group of people comes to be seen as a threat to social values and interests (Cohen, 1972). These panics are driven by a constellation of 'moral entrepreneurs' who play a key role in defining the crisis through their interest-based claims-making (Cohen, 1972; Showalter, 1997). For more on obesity and moral panics see LeBesco (2010).

Though there are many potential lines of analysis related to obesity and US media, and an almost infinite number of media representations of obesity to draw on and explore, in this chapter, I broadly present what I see as the main themes characterizing media treatment of obesity in the first decade of the epidemic and which have continued to define media coverage of obesity through the last decade. I then consider what these general themes, taken together, can tell us not only about obesity in the United States, but, more significantly, about the social, cultural, and economic interests and anxieties that undergird and perpetuate the US obsession with obesity. I conclude with a discussion of potential new avenues of scholarship on obesity in the media, particularly as media become more interactive and less tied to traditional forms of print and television dissemination.

This analysis relies primarily on news articles on obesity appearing in *The New York Times* between 1990 and 2011. *The New York Times* reporting on obesity does not represent a comprehensive picture of the media's approach to the obesity epidemic.[2] Yet, I have chosen *The New York Times* coverage of obesity for three reasons (Boero, 2007; 2012). First, the 'obesity epidemic' has been portrayed as a national crisis of major significance and it is only fitting that a study of this epidemic should rely on a leading national news source. *The New York Times* is a leading opinion centre and setter among intellectuals, professionals, policy makers and the general educated public (Gitlin, 1980). Second, *The New York Times* is noted for its science writing and many of the contradictions and complexities of this epidemic orbit around perceptions of science and medicine.[3] Third, as the transmission of medical and scientific knowledge expands beyond the clinic to health-related information via the media and the internet, sources like *The New York Times* become more central to the layperson's understanding of health, science, and medicine (Conrad, 2007; Barker, 2005; Clarke et al., 2003).

In this chapter, I will focus on three main themes that emerge in this coverage, themes that have been consistently present in media discussions of obesity since the early 1990s. The first theme is that of obesity as a threat to the fiscal and physical health of the United States. In an era where health care expenditures continue to soar, obesity has been portrayed as one of the major culprits in the increasing costs of medical care. Yet the culprit status of obesity is not limited to the health care arena, and it is notable that the growing prevalence of obesity has been blamed for processes as disparate as climate change and the rising costs

2 Prior to the emergence of the 'obesity epidemic' as an object of concern, weight and weight-loss were seen as the terrain of women and the vast majority of media coverage of these and related topics appeared in publications specifically marketed to women. Feminist scholars have long criticized the mainstream media for their role in creating and perpetuating unattainable and ethnocentric ideals of health and beauty. See Gruys (2013), Bordo (1993) and Chernin (1981) for a further discussion of women's magazines and the culture of thinness.

3 I and others have written more extensively on the representation of the science of obesity in the media elsewhere (Boero, 2007; 2012; Saguy & Almeling, 2008).

of airline travel. Second, I will look at how the purported negative health effects of obesity are presented as both scientific fact and also as common sense. I will suggest that, as we move into the third decade of the 'obesity epidemic', it becomes evident that what we now (supposedly) know about fatness and fat people from a scientific perspective is nearly indistinguishable from what we have 'known' for decades (or more) about fatness and fat people from a moral perspective. Third, I will look at how, especially in the last 10 years, obesity has come to be presented in the media as primarily an affliction of the poor, minorities, and children. Indeed, it is these groups who are not only the focus of much of recent media coverage of obesity, but are also most intensively targeted by growing numbers of anti-obesity policy initiatives. I will conclude by considering the functions and consequences of the constant re-iteration of these themes for the past 20 years.[4]

Obesity is a Problem that Threatens the Physical and Fiscal Health of the United States

The first overarching theme found in media reporting on the 'obesity epidemic' is that fatness is a danger to individual and public health. Related to this, obesity is viewed as an economic threat to US society, not only in terms of public health spending but also in terms of military readiness. Articles that fall within this theme most often focus on three intersecting areas: obesity as a crisis, the current and projected future costs of obesity, and the causes of and potential cures for obesity.

Two quotes, one from 1994 and the other from 2006, illustrate the media's persistent focus on obesity as a crisis. In the first quote, excerpted from his editorial in the *Journal of the American Medical Association*, obesity researcher Dr F. Xavier Pi Sunyer asserts, 'The proportion of the population that is obese is incredible. If this was about tuberculosis, it would be called an epidemic' (Burros, 1994). Although it is now commonplace to speak of an 'obesity epidemic', this quote marks one of the first times obesity is referred to as an 'epidemic' in the mainstream media. Twelve years later, the focus on the urgency of obesity as not only a public health issue but also as an issue of national security comes through in this statement from former United States Surgeon General Dr Richard Carmona when he declared, 'Obesity is the terror within. Unless we do something about it, the magnitude of the dilemma will dwarf 9/11 or any other terrorist attempt'[5] (Associated Press, 2006). This second quote clearly reflects the post 9/11 intensification of the language of threat and risk by both public officials and the

4 Some of the data and themes presented in this chapter appeared in an earlier article on obesity in the US from 1990–2001 media, published in the journal *Qualitative Sociology* (Boero, 2007). However, in this chapter, I expand my analysis to discuss media coverage of obesity from 2001 through 2011.

5 See also Biltekoff (2007); Saguy & Almeling (2008).

media. These two quotes from *The New York Times* and the Associated Press, while separated by more than a decade, are both intended to convey the urgency surrounding 'epidemic' obesity.

Much of the urgency surrounding obesity comes from a significant oversight in media coverage of the rates of obesity. In 1998, the United States National Institutes of Health (NIH) officially lowered the BMI threshold for both obesity and overweight.[6] This measure was aligned with recommendations for the international standardization of BMI indicators (Shetty & James, 1994); however, as a result of the NIH decision, overnight, 50 million more Americans entered the ranks of the overweight and obese without gaining a single ounce. Significantly, this change allowed the media and public health officials to say that more than half of Americans were either overweight or obese. Nowhere in *The New York Times* was this shift in BMI threshold mentioned as being, in part, responsible for the rapid rise in rates of overweight and obesity observed in the late 1990s.[7]

In the media, numbers are central to conveying a sense of urgency around various social problems from crime to teenage pregnancy and school drop-out rates. Like the de-contextualized statistics on rates of obesity, ongoing attempts to put both a price and a death toll on obesity are part and parcel of media coverage of obesity. For example, in a 1998 article, *New York Times* contributor Gina Kolata cites a claim made by a former US surgeon general and his colleagues about the numbers of deaths *caused* by obesity – 'obesity causes 318,000 excess deaths a year' – without detailing how these numbers were calculated. As many authors have pointed out, in the case of reporting on obesity, cause and correlation are frequently confounded, particularly when calculating the supposed number of obesity-related deaths and the purported financial costs of obesity (Campos, 2004; Oliver, 2005; Saguy, 2013). More than ten years after the article cited above was published, *The New York Times* continues to publish statistics on obesity that offer little information on how they are calculated but which do provide moralistic commentary that often squares with readers' preconceived notions about the eating habits of larger people. In an article on the health and economic costs of obesity, Jane Brody reports that,

---

6 BMI does not actually measure body fat but rather the relationship between weight and height. Prior to 1998, 'overweight' was considered to be a BMI greater than or equal to 27.8 in men and 27.0 for women. In 1998, the National Institutes of Health (NIH) made the decision to lower the BMI threshold for 'overweight' to 25 and for 'obesity' to a BMI greater than or equal to 30 for all people regardless of sex or body fat composition, thus greatly increasing the number of Americans falling into both categories of 'overweight' and 'obese'. Some estimates suggest that this change caused more than 30 million Americans to move from normal to overweight overnight (Hubbard, 2000).

7 As many have pointed out, in spite of criticism, the BMI remains the default measure of obesity largely because it is a single, easily calculable number. For criticism of the BMI, see Boero (2012), Holland et al. (2011), Oliver (2005), Campos (2004).

> Together, the added treatment costs of obesity, already at $75 billion in 2003, could exceed $66 billion a year, with an even greater cost in lost productivity of up to $580 billion. The cancer statistics alone should be enough to keep one's mouth from closing on a double cheeseburger and fries. (Brody, 2011)

This second quote points to another central focus of articles that emphasize obesity as a social crisis, namely an implicit or explicit focus on the causes and 'cures' for obesity. By suggesting that simply avoiding burgers and french fries is enough to avoid supposedly obesity-related cancers, Kolata implies that in spite of the multifactorial causes of rising weights, weight gain is really a simple consequence of poor eating habits. Indeed, while a number of 'causes' of obesity, ranging from genetic to environmental to cultural, are occasionally explored in *The New York Times*, even in the various articles that appear to advocate for these less individualistic explanations, individual behaviour is always returned to as the most significant explanation of rising US weights. In a 1997 article about possible viral explanations for obesity, the final line reads: 'Poor diet and lack of exercise are the overwhelming causes of obesity, doctors agree' (Anon, 1997). Thus, what we feel we know about the eating habits and lifestyles of fat people becomes taken-for-granted in media reporting on weight-related issues.

The Obesity Epidemic and the Negative Health Impacts of Obesity are both Scientific Givens and Common Sense

The media's reiteration of contested numbers on the economic and physical costs of obesity, along with the assumption that overweight and obesity are necessarily unhealthy and solely the result of individual habits, construct the 'obesity epidemic' as a scientific given that can nonetheless be verified through simple common sense. The US media, including *The New York Times*, present the obesity epidemic as a scientific fact and body mass index as a reliable measure of both body composition and overall health. While a small percentage of *The New York Times* reporting on obesity does question some of the claims made about the link between weight and health, nowhere does *The New York Times* question the existence of the epidemic. Even reports that question some received knowledge about fatness, fat people, and dieting fall far short of critically interrogating the very existence of the epidemic. And more often than not end up pointing to the dangers of not taking obesity seriously.

Two articles in *The New York Times* illustrate this well. The first article takes on the marketing of fraudulent diet products and another article is about those who fight medical, employment, and social discrimination against fat people. However, neither of these two articles questions the science or undesirability of fatness even as the latter seeks to debunk some of the more common myths about fat people themselves.

In the first article, by Gina Kolata (2000), entitled, 'How the Body Knows When to Gain or Lose', Kolata reports on findings connecting deficiencies in the hormone leptin with increasing weight. The article features an interview with Dr Jeffrey Friedman, a researcher who studies leptin and weight. Dr Friedman suggests that it is a complex balance of genes, hormones, and brain signals that determines a person's weight range, not individual behaviours. Following from this, Dr Friedman says that traditional weight-loss diets are virtually doomed to failure because weight is largely outside of an individual's control. Kolata also reports that these developments in the science of obesity have been of interest not only to overweight people tired of constantly failing at diets but also to pharmaceutical companies hoping these early discoveries might lead to blockbuster weight-loss drugs. Dr Friedman and other obesity researchers quoted in the article adhere to a disease model of obesity and are optimistic about the development of medical interventions for obesity. Dr Gregory Barsh, a Stanford University researcher hopes to re-frame obesity as a disease: 'There's been a prejudice, a bias that obesity is a behavioral abnormality … somehow in the past, obesity was thought of as a poor relation to a real disease like heart disease or cancer. This misperception is being corrected' (Kolata, 2000). The idea of a genetic or hormonal basis to the epidemic is compelling in its potential to take the blame for fatness off of individuals and provide hope for a medical solution to the epidemic. It is notable, however, that this article was one in a series that included an article on 'extreme surgical treatment for weight loss', underscoring how the medicalization of obesity aetiology, while potentially legitimizing for those labelled obese, can also justify potentially dangerous and invasive interventions such as bariatric surgeries and poorly tested pharmaceuticals for weight loss. Moreover, the article itself does not question the existence of the epidemic, dominant ideas about the relationship between weight and health, or the desirability and importance of weight-loss.

The second article, 'Fat but Fit', by Jane Brody (2000), presents the cases of several people who feel themselves to be both fat and fit, including Dr Steven Blair, a fitness researcher at the Cooper Institute in Dallas, TX. Blair and others have found that overweight and obese people who eat a low-fat diet and exercise increase their fitness levels and lower their risk for certain conditions even as they remain overweight. They have also found that fat and fit people have a lower death risk than thin people who are sedentary. This article stands out in the abundance of reporting on the dangers and costs of obesity for challenging the automatic association of fatness with lack of fitness and conversely the assumption that thin people are healthy regardless of fitness levels. Yet again, the article does not challenge the idea that ultimately being fat is bad and unhealthy. After telling the story of Cheryl Haworth, a 300-pound Olympic weight lifter who can also do the splits, Brody cautions, 'This does not mean it is O.K. to be overweight. A person who is lean and fit still does better in terms of health than someone who is fit but remains fat. But while everyone can't become lean, becoming fit is possible for anyone willing to make the effort'. Thus, thinness is still the gold standard of health and obesity remains a threat to health even for those willing to take on the challenge of becoming fit.

Using the existence of the 'obesity epidemic' as a taken-for-granted starting point for reporting on obesity has the effect of silencing critical voices and training media focus on intervention into and prevention of obesity, rather than on larger discussions about public health. The sheer volume of media attention to obesity points to the fact that the 'obesity epidemic' is not just a concern or product of discussions among policy makers and government officials. Indeed, this media dissemination of the purported *scientific facts* about weight and health reflects and reproduces what has become our larger *common-sense knowledge* about weight such that we are all becoming obesity experts. It is easy for the media to tap into what we have long thought we already know about fatness, fat people, and health (Boero, 2007; 2012).

Obesity as an Affliction of the Poor, Children, and Minorities

In the early 1990s, most discussions of obesity focused on overall obesity rates, sometimes broken down by sex or age. But, with the collection of more health data that include racial and ethnic identification and income, the higher than average obesity rates among some portions of the US population are targeted as being particularly problematic, namely, African Americans, Hispanics, children, and the poor. A 'culture of obesity' has come to be the default explanation for rising weights among these populations. Yet, as I have argued elsewhere (Boero, 2007; 2012), this 'culture of obesity' refers to culture in two different senses. The first usage of culture is illustrated by the two quotes below and generally refers to American 'convenience culture' – a culture of fast-food, 'labour saving devices', and sedentary lifestyle.

> We live in a toxic environment with regard to obesity. Food is very palatable, very cheap, very easy to get. Labor saving devices are everywhere. Everybody is working at desks, expending a lot less energy and eating a lot more. (Freudenheim, 1999)

> If the child learns to eat from their overweight parent, who learned from their overweight parent, and Mom buys the same way and does the same thing she did years ago, and now that kid isn't even running and jumping the way kids used to, that child is in trouble. (Lombardi, 1997)

These two quotes represent the tendency of the US media to point to larger trends in US culture without much attention to how these trends in employment, activity level and food production, distribution, preparation, and consumption are not spread evenly throughout the US populace. Indeed, this lack of context extends even further when the media discuss rising weights among particular racial and ethnic groups. This comes through most clearly in articles discussing the food preparation and eating habits of racial and ethnic subcultures and how these practices may be contributing to the 'obesity epidemic' in minority communities. This comes across clearly in 'Why baked catfish holds lessons for their heart', an article in *The New York Times* detailing a programme implemented in a small southern town by researchers from the University of Alabama (Marcus, 1998). The programme targets African American food practices in the rural south, an area in which a fatty diet predates the Civil War and is said to represent the most extreme contemporary example of 'a nutritionist's bad dream'. The article describes a community in which,

> ... there are three doctors, no hospitals, no ambulances, no 911 services ... The population is 79 percent African-American; the jobless rate is edging towards 14 percent and the median family income is $12,497 ... Browse the shelves: along with ingredients for Southern staples like corn bread and fried chicken stretches a range of pig parts from head to foot, including brains and fatty ham hocks and tails. Pork chitterlings for frying are available in ten-pound buckets; fatback by the slab and fatty beef parts are popular, too. Lard flies off the shelves in eight-pound cans. (Marcus, 1998)

According to *The New York Times*, programme leaders are attempting to improve community health by 'teaching women how to stay well by changing their behavior ... and doing the unthinkable – banishing collard greens smothered in fatback and other traditional high-fat favorites in the rural South' (Marcus, 1998). This is but one example of the targeting of African American and Hispanic communities to the effect that we now have a 'culture of obesity' framework that works much the same way culture of poverty arguments did in the 1960s – to blame people for their own ill-health and poverty and to shift attention away from structural inequalities.

Conclusion

Taken together, these three broad themes in US media coverage of obesity reveal three intersecting patterns. First, in a society that is uncomfortable talking about poverty, race, and ethnicity, obesity has become a way to talk about all three, often in conjunction, without ever discussing larger structures and patterns of inequality. This is especially true when we see wealth and income inequality at an all-time high, quality medical care becoming less and less accessible, and a social safety net that continues to shrink. Second, these themes point to the current and growing equation of health with morality in which the care of the self becomes the project of public health (Lupton, 1999; Metzel & Kirkland, 2010).[8] Finally, media coverage of obesity fits with the needs of both public health agencies and diet industry profiteers to individualize ill health and move focus from inequality to personal behaviour and cultural practices (Boero, 2012).

Obesity continues to be framed in the media as a problem of individual habits or will. Yet as more and more attention to obesity comes to be focused on particular population subsets (such as the poor, children, etc.), it is likely that policy will come to reflect media framings of fatness in these particular groups as well as pre-existing frames of these groups more generally (Campo and Mastin, 2007; Boero, 2010). For example, the framing of children as impressionable and innocent drives childhood obesity policy that focuses on television advertising of 'junk' food and banning toys in fast food meals for children (Udell and Mehta, 2008). It is unlikely that these same sorts of approaches would be taken with policies aimed at adults who are seen as much more culpable for their own and their children's health. Nonetheless, the framings of both childhood and adult obesity ignore the structural conditions under which people live.

A focus on the relationship between media portrayals of obesity and specific policy initiatives is a relatively new area of inquiry. However, as scholars of obesity and media have pointed out, in limiting our framings of obesity in the media to those discussed above, we potentially limit the scope of our policy in ways that preclude addressing wider social inequities in health and health care. A narrow focus on obesity as a health problem, combined with its framing as an individual problem, effectively closes off discussions of health that focus on the relationship between weight, poverty, access to care, stigma, discrimination, race, gender, and overall wellness (Rothblum, 1999; Boero, 2007; 2012; 2013).

There is no doubt that the amount of media attention to obesity will continue to grow as researchers secure more funding to come up with solutions, as more obesity policy is debated and enacted, and as governments continue to individualize responsibility for public health. The task of social scientists will be not only to keep up with this reporting but also to sharpen their critical focus. This can happen by bringing in more voices and not only pointing out that the media marginalize alternative framings of obesity, but actually elaborating and highlighting some of those silenced interpretations that move beyond simple equations of weight and social and economic crisis. Media analysts need to take a lead in deconstructing the taken-for-granted – in this case, the 'obesity epidemic'.

---

8 In her study of media coverage of obesity since 2001, Helene Shugart (2011) suggests that predominant earlier frames of obesity as a result of either environmental factors *or* individual behaviours have been supplanted by a fatalistic framing in which obesity is seen to be both unavoidable and inevitable. Shugart suggests that this fatalism supersedes the binary framing of obesity as a result of environmental factors or individual behaviours but that this fatalism does not reduce stigma against fat people or encourage further discussion of the social determinants of health, rather it forecloses a more complex discussion of weight and health (Shugart, 2011; Boero, 2013).

References

Anon (1997, April 8). Virus may lie behind some obesity. *The New York Times*. Retrieved from www.nytimes.com

Associated Press (2006, March 2). Surgeon general: Obesity epidemic will dwarf terrorism threat. *Health SciTech*.

Barker, K. (2005). *The fibromyalgia story: Biomedical authority and women's worlds of pain*. Nashville: Vanderbilt University Press.

Biltekoff, C. (2007). The terror within: Obesity in post 9/11 US life. *American Studies, 48(3)*, 29–48.

Boero, N. (2007). All the news that's fat to print: The American 'obesity epidemic' and the media. *Qualitative Sociology, 30(1)*, 41–60

Boero, N. (2009). Fat kids working moms and the 'epidemic of obesity': Race, class, and mother blame. In E. Rothblum & S. Solovay (eds), *The fat studies reader* (pp. 113–120). New York: New York University Press.

Boero, N. (2012). *Killer fat: Media, medicine and morals in the American 'obesity epidemic'*. New Brunswick: Rutgers University Press.

Boero, N. (2013). Obesity and the media: Social science weighs in. *Critical Public Health, 23(3)*, 371–380.

Bordo, S. (1993). *Unbearable weight: Feminism, western culture, and the body*. Berkeley: University of California Press.

Brody, J. (2000). Fat but fit: A myth about obesity is slowly being debunked. *The New York Times*. Retrieved from www.nytimes.com

Brody, J. (2011, September 12). The numbers behind an urgent fight. *The New York Times*. Retrieved from www.nytimes.com

Burros, M. (1994, July 17). Despite awareness of risks, more in U.S. are getting fat. *The New York Times*. Retrieved from www.nytimes.com

Campos, P. (2004). *The obesity myth: Why America's obsession with weight is hazardous for your health*. New York: Gotham Books.

Chernin, K. (1994). *The hungry self: Women, eating, and identity*. New York: Harper Perennial.

Clarke, A., Shim, J., Mamo, L., et al. (2003). Biomedicalization: Technoscientific transformations of health, illness, and U.S. biomedicine. *American Sociological Review, 68*, 161–194.

Cohen, S. (1972). *Folk devils and moral panics*. New York: Routledge.

Conrad, P. (2007). *The medicalization of society: On the transformation of human conditions into treatable disorders*. Baltimore: Johns Hopkins University Press.

Freudenheim, M. (1999, September 6). Employers focus on weight as workplace health issue. *The New York Times*. Retrieved from www.nytimes.com

Gard, M. & Wright, J. (2005). *The obesity epidemic: Science, morality, and ideology*. New York: Routledge.

Gitlin. T. (1980). *The whole world is watching: Mass media in the making & unmaking of the New Left*. Berkeley: University of California Press.

Glassner, B. (2000). *The culture of fear: Why Americans are afraid of the wrong things*. New York: Basic Books.

Goode, E. & Ben-Yehuda, N. (1994). *Moral panics: The social construction of deviance*. Oxford: Blackwell.

Gruys, K. (2013). *Mirror, mirror off the wall: How I learned to love my body by not looking at it for a year.* New York. Avery.

Holland, K., Blood, R., Thomas, S., et al. (2011). 'Our girth is plain to see': An analysis of newspaper coverage of Australia's future 'fat bomb'. *Health, Risk & Society, 13(1)*, 31–46.

Kolata, G. (1998, January 11). The nation: Not quite seconds for everyone; the fat's in the fire, again. *The New York Times*. Retrieved from www.nytimes.com

Kolata, G. (2000, October 17). How the body knows how to gain or lose. *The New York Times*. Retrieved from www.nytimes.com

LeBesco, K. (2010). Fat panic and the new morality. In A. Kirkland & J. Metzl (eds), *Against health: How health became the new morality* (pp. 72–83). New York: New York University Press.

Lombardi, K.S. (1997). Treating child obesity: From healthy eating to working out. *The New York Times*. Retrieved from www.nytimes.com

Lupton, D. (1999). *Risk*. New York. Routledge.

Marcus, F.F. (1998, June 21). Why baked catfish holds lessons for their hearts. *The New York Times*. Retrieved from www.nytimes.com

Mastin, T. & Campo, S. (2006). Conflicting messages: Overweight and obesity advertisements and articles in black magazines. *The Howard Journal of Communications, 17(4)*, 265–285.

Metzl, J. & Kirkland, A. (2010). *Against health: How health became the new morality.* New York: New York University Press.

Oliver, J.E. (2006). *Fat politics: The real story behind America's obesity epidemic.* New York: Oxford University Press.

Rothblum, E. (1999). Contradictions and confounds in coverage of obesity: Psychology journals, textbooks, and the media. *Journal of Social Issues, 55(2)*, 355–369.

Saguy, A. (2013). *What's wrong with fat?* New York. Oxford University Press.

Saguy, A. & Almeling, R. (2008). Fat in the fire? Science, the news media, and the 'obesity epidemic'. *Sociological Forum, 23(1)*, 53–83.

Saguy, A. & Gruys, K. (2010). Morality and health: News media constructions of overweight and eating disorders. *Social Problems, 57(2)*, 231–50.

Saguy, A., Gruys, K. & Gong, S. (2010). Social problem construction and national context: News reporting on 'Overweight' and 'Obesity' in the United States and France. *Social Problems, 57(4)*, 586–610.

Shetty, P.S. & James, W.P.T. (1994). Body mass index: A measure of chronic energy deficiency in adults. *FAO Food and Nutrition Paper*, 56.

Showalter, E. (1997). *Hystories: Hysterical epidemics and modern media.* New York: Columbia University Press.

Shugart, H. (2011). Heavy viewing: Emergent frames in contemporary news coverage of obesity. *Health Communication*, *26*, 635–648.

Udell, T. & Mehta, K. (2008). When two sides go to war: Newspaper reporting of television food advertising restrictions' as a solution to childhood obesity. *Health, Risk & Society*, *10(6)*, 535–548.

Chapter 4

Invisible Fat: The Aesthetics of Food and the Body

Pino Donghi and Josephine Wennerholm

Introduction

From the end of World War II, standards of living improved dramatically across the Western world. Evidence for rapidly rising obesity rates has come from regular, nationally representative surveys from the 1960s onwards, but it was not until the 1980s that public awareness of the issue became apparent, with the help of the media (Caballero, 2007). If the 1980s mark the timing of onset of public disquiet about body fatness, they also mark significant change in the political climate, with the fall of Communism, the coming to power of Ronald Reagan and Margaret Thatcher in the United States and the United Kingdom, and the neoliberal economic paradigms that spread from these countries. This new climate upheld the importance of an aesthetically pleasing body (most commonly thin and fit) as a sign of good health and consequently ushered in attendant elitist social mores, while appealing to other cultural shifts in the structuring of domestic and social realms, and in particular, women's roles therein. The spread of this aesthetic could not have happened so quickly or widely across the Western world without the aid of mass media (film and television) and technological advances in communication (the advent of internet and mobile telephones). All this took place while obesity rates soared. The rise in obesity could not have taken place without the food industry promoting lifestyles in the fast lane, with convenient, packaged and fast foods available all day long, all year round and at low cost. Such lifestyles in neoliberal economies have involved increased personal stress levels, with working hours increasing to the extent that many people perceive themselves as not having enough time to cook. The food industry has been able to thrive in such consumer-driven societies because it can steer advertising to promote its products as 'part of the solution', pandering either to the fear-mongering associated with health issues, or to people's need to pamper themselves and their desire for the superfluous. And while popular news media accounts now frame anorexia compassionately (Ferris, 2003; Saguy & Gruys, 2010), the obese person still comes across as lacking in self-discipline, despite growing evidence of a strong link between stress and weight gain (Offer et al., 2010).

This chapter examines the parallels between the visual templates of foods and bodies, as they appear in a number of media. It explores the aesthetic and moral models implied by the images they create, use and disseminate, with particular attention to the visual linking of 'fat free' foods and bodies, with beauty, cleanliness and moral obligation as conceived in a neoliberal context.

Culinary Beauty

In *History of Beauty*, Eco (2004) poses the question: what ideal of beauty has prevailed at different times across the ages? Eco courses chronologically through various historical periods, linking different beauty ideals with each, be it Ancient Greece, the Renaissance, or the modern era. A common thread is the illustration of a 'unifying trait' for each era, a fundamental characteristic that can stand out and be identifiable as representative of the historical period in question, one that can clearly outline the dominant aesthetic. When it comes to the twentieth century, Eco maintains that it is beyond him to define any unifying trait, even though he cannot rule out the possibility that the hypothetical future art historian or space traveller might instead be able to pinpoint one with the benefit of distance. So far as the first half of the twentieth century is concerned, and maybe even up to the 1960s, all we can do for now, says Eco, is make do with the idea that this time frame saw the battle between 'Beauty as provocation and Beauty as consumerism' (2004: 16).

The ideals of 'beauty as provocation' can be found in the avant-garde art movements of futurism, cubism, expressionism and surrealism. Rather than concentrating on the problem of Beauty, members of such art movements wanted to explore how the world could be interpreted from different perspectives, even when they were drawing on archaic or exotic models. The exception to this was abstraction, which relied heavily on geometric harmony, going back to Classical Greece and the many neoclassical movements that followed. Eco uses the device of space-time travellers, who peer into different periods and discover novelties that perhaps someone closer to the people and the phenomena observed would not. In the case of the middle and late twentieth century, Eco's space-time travellers might encounter groups of people visiting an avant-garde exhibition. These people may buy a statue that is 'incomprehensible' to them, or take part in a 'happening'. And while participating in avant-garde activities:

> they will be dressed and coiffed according to the canons of fashion, wearing jeans or designer label clothes as well as make-up that have all been proposed as the model of Beauty by glossy magazines, the cinema and television, i.e. by the mass media. They follow the ideals of Beauty that are propounded by the bastion of market consumerism, the very bastion that avant garde art movements have been fighting against for more than fifty years. (2010: 418)

According to Eco, this is the typical contradiction of the twentieth century.

Beauty as consumerism has its roots in the emergent fashion advertising of the late nineteenth century, when women's magazines began to circulate more widely, and in the early twentieth century, when fashion plates allowed the greater mass circulation of female bodily ideals (Stewart & Janovicek, 2001). Both of these promoted thinness to the elite, with the associated encouragement of fitness to reduce body fatness (Stewart & Janovicek, 2001). By 1890, thinness had become a way in which young privileged women in the United States and Europe could distinguish themselves from their working-class counterparts (Brumberg, 1988). Even before the emergence of the flapper in the 1920s, the struggle for bodily thinness among American women was underway, and was taken very personally (Brumberg, 1988). Hollywood, and the film industry more generally, took this struggle to the masses. It created a cast of 'stars' who were to be adored from afar but could be viewed very closely on the screen. The movies were affordable by all and, unlike art movements, exhibitions, or magazines, were not elitist. Hollywood went to great lengths to create a modern-day 'Olympus of Gods' for the mortals going to the movies to admire and emulate; magazine and newspaper media facilitated this process by concocting stories about these actor-gods in 'real-life' and set the fashions of the day through the movies. Films were promoted as the stuff of which dreams are made and could be relied on to give a strong visual base from which taste and fashion could be shaped. This was an era where censorship, Christian morality and ideas of classical beauty still held sway, however, and standards of appearance and behaviour still had to be maintained. This God-like world began to unravel from the late fifties onwards, when the hierarchical Hollywood star system began to decline with the rise of television and its more down-to-earth offering of on-screen viewings at home, eventually across the day. The idea of a lean and fit body as a prerequisite of beauty, as a way of 'packaging' the human body to ensure attractiveness as well as longevity, percolated into the media by the 1980s, with an emergent industry around self-improvement, in which exposure to bodily ideals became everyday, inside the home as well as without. Associated with this was an ideology of limitless improvement and change, defying the historicity, the mortality, and, often, the very materiality of the body itself (Bordo, 1993).

Yet, at this intersection of body and consumerist ideals, there is another, perhaps less obvious, materiality governed by beauty: food. Eating is shaped by cultural boundaries and frames that may appear as tacit guidelines or strictures from within but are really expressions of ethnic, religious or social group practices (Bourdieu, 1977). When it comes to nutrition, necessity, aesthetics, and ethics cannot be separated. The aesthetics of food have shaped subsistence and feeding practices from prehistoric times (Farringdon & Urry, 1985) to the present. In recent times, the nouvelle cuisine of the 1970s in France set off a fashion for food presentation that shows no sign of slacking, at least in higher end restaurants. However, cuisine has been 'nouvelling' itself, at least since the middle of the eighteenth century in France, with food fads, fashions and trends emerging and varying according to the availability of means, resourcefulness, creativity, and the power of dissemination (Mennel, 1986; Elias, 1978). Food need not always have an aesthetic appeal, but the receptacle of food – our body with its external indication of good health – most definitely does.

Imagining the Body, Marketing Food

While the linking of beauty to the lean and fit body has deep roots in the history of Western thought, in the United States and Europe, the democratic dissemination of this ideal, together with the new industry of self-improvement, took off only three decades ago. What is also relatively new is the public disapproval of 'fat' in all its forms, be it in the physical body or in food. In many countries, the food industry has adopted and amplified this trend, making so-called low fat foods very convenient to buy and consume, and advertising them as the 'smart' thing to consume, particularly through televised commercials.

Television entered as a fixture in nearly all homes in the West by the 1960s. Television broadcasting, especially in the United States, was not discrete from commercial interest. Reithian principles of broadcasting (which are to inform, educate and entertain) could not compete with the free-market approach to broadcasting, where programming was thought out in terms of attracting the largest audiences or advertising revenues. Television thus became an ideal channel for advertising and setting new trends in food consumption too. With an emphasis on the embellishment of packaged food, the age of stimulated appetite had arrived:

> The hugely intensified expectation of tastiness and pleasing appearance that typifies our post-industrial gastronomic culture is clearly expressed in packaging design ... Colourings and taste enhancers developed in laboratories are designed primarily to stimulate the appetite (not to be confused with biological hunger) of the consumer, and hence increase the marketability of the product. (Teuteberg 2007: 260)

When appetite cannot be satisfied according to nutritional need, it can lead to unexpected dietary preferences or choices. Dickson Wright (2012) illustrates this using George Orwell's words, on poverty and unemployment in Britain during the early 1930s:

> This is the era of George Orwell's The Road to Wigan Pier, and his account is perhaps the most vivid of those seeking to explain what life was like for those struggling against poverty. People by now could claim some state assistance, but it was never enough to keep a family well fed and housed. Orwell describes an unemployed miner's family trying to get by on a diet that essentially consisted of white bread and margarine, corned beef, sugared tea and potatoes. He also makes a very telling point about the diet of the poor. Some, he argues, would suggest that rather than waste money on such non-essentials as tea and sugar, it would be healthier for the unemployed to buy fresh oranges and raw carrots:
>
> Yes, it would, but the point is that no ordinary human being is ever going to do such a thing. The ordinary human being would sooner starve than live on brown bread and raw carrots. And the peculiar evil is this, that the less money you

> have, the less inclined you feel to spend it on wholesome food. A millionaire may enjoy breakfasting off orange juice and Ryvita biscuits; an unemployed doesn't. (2012: 413–414)

Orwell, paraphrased by Dickson Wright, goes on to explain why the poor so often eat junk food: it's easy and it's comforting.

> Let's have a three pennorth of chips! Run out and buy us a twopenny ice-cream! Put the kettle on and we'll have a nice cup of tea! To condemn them for this is to misunderstand what poverty is like. (2012: 414)

The modern food industry *does* understand (and indeed has to understand) these dynamics to produce targeted packaging and messaging, with appeal and convenience for its particular markets, rich and poor, regardless of the nutritional contents of the foods it promotes. A lot of research goes into the presentation of junk food – the food may be of limited nutritional value for good health but it still has to be presented and displayed in attractive ways and priced to maximize sales.

Packaging of food and packaging of the body go together. Among other things, packaging and marketing are about promoting *lifestyles* of consumption (Baudrillard, 2007 [1970]), and pandering to common human desires beyond the need for survival. And the desire for perfect bodies is seemingly endless, as evidenced by the industries of fitness, cosmetics, cosmetic surgery, slimming, fashion and media, regardless of health imperatives, gender, and age.

The powerfully athletic and youthfully packaged fit thin body is what now serves as a marker of social status and cultural capital (Ulijaszek, 2012). In parallel with this, food magazines or images have come to feature the single plate of food (as opposed to the serving dish or platter) as the cynosure for conspicuous consumption. Thanks to the efforts and work of French chefs and to the nouvelle cuisine they launched, the appearance of food on the plate took on greater importance than ever before. This aesthetic was inspired by Japanese chefs and their rich and artistic tradition of serving food (according to Richard Hosking [1996: 209], chefs might 'spend the day considering the aesthetics of arranging three sardines'). Beautiful china plates and formal dinner table sets gave way to the single, pure white and very large plate, to train the eye on the object at hand, the artistically arranged food. In Michel Guérard's *Cuisine Minceur* (1977), all recipes were low calorie versions for nouvelle cuisine. The implication was that the old, fat gourmand was dead: Long Live the new, slim gastronome, and hey! you can have your cake and eat it too.

Elitist eating lost some of its conviviality in this zeitgeist, as well as some of its socializing function. The emphasis was on the 'experience' of eating beautiful food and recognizing the evanescence of its nature or its role in keeping the body healthy and 'naturally' slim. This type of cooking seemed easy and was therefore copied – but it was copied badly. It could not function in the world of 'ordinary' people unless eateries descended from their pedestal and walked among the people, which they did, according to Wells (2000): 'The modern American restaurant seduces its audience with movie-set design, stage lighting, celebrity chefs and themed menus. Like many other things in this country, restaurants are a branch of the entertainment industry'. The trend may have started in the United States but spread quickly enough. Where once the kitchen was to be kept out of sight of diners and dinner-table guests, it now became centre stage. Food programmes on television spread like a rash, many audience-members imagining themselves to be able to cook like a celebrity chef someday. The dish being prepared on the TV screen might be touted as being 'simple' to make, but cookery programmes are steeped in ostentatious showmanship and one-upmanship to maintain their audience-pulling attraction.

While fast food restaurants had their origins in the 1920s, their expansion came in the 1960s with economic prosperity and the emergence of other symbols of modernism, including supermarkets, frozen foods and convenience meals. The fast-food industry grew in parallel with the penetration of television into all corners of American life, eventually locating fast food restaurants and services at the centre of all major towns, cities, new housing developments and major transport hubs. In cinemas, fast food could be eaten while the fit thin bodies of movie stars could be admired.

The Moving Images of Consumption

With cooking no longer conceived as a social necessity, and with new foods and ingredients flooding supermarkets, photo spreads and television programmes, media food presentation acquired a pornographic element. In the making of her film *Julie and Julia*, the late Nora Ephron (2010) specifically asked her cameraman to film the dishes in a 'pornographic' manner. The pornographication of food by the popular media has been discussed by O'Neill (2003) and Magee (2007). O'Neill (2003) has defined food pornography as food writing or imagery that is removed from real life, and Magee (2003) adds to this definition by stressing the voyeurism attached to the witnessing of food preparation in the media. Thus, food, when removed from the kitchen, becomes divorced from its nutritive or taste qualities and enters a realm where surface appearance is all-important (Magee, 2007). Media chefs have become commodity celebrities (Brownlee & Hewer, 2009) fuelling food desires beyond those of mere sustenance.

Roland Barthes (2009 [1957]) picked up on the mythic aspects of food spreads in magazines over half a century ago, targeting 'Ornamental Cookery' in one of his *Mythologies* essays written between 1954 and 1956. The colour photographs in *Elle* magazine sold a 'dream of smartness' to the working class, he wrote (2009:89). Shown from a high angle, at once near and inaccessible, the food could be consumed 'simply by looking' by people who could dream of partridges but not afford them. Any actual food was 'no more than an indeterminate bed-rock' beneath 'sedimentary layers' of smooth 'coatings and alibis' (2009: 89). For the 'primary nature of foodstuffs, the brutality of meat or the abruptness of seafood' was buried beneath sauces, creams, icing and jellies (2009: 89). These coverings were the blank page for a 'fairy-land reality' of chiselled mushrooms, carved lemons, shavings of truffle, and arabesques of *glacé* fruit (2009: 91). Barthes knows and says that the onlookers have trouble affording these foods. This is elegant parlance for saying people are hoodwinked. They are being side-tracked by ornamental cookery from dwelling on more important life challenges.

The cultures of body enhancement and contemporary eating behaviours among the privileged are linked. When food is cheap, it is easier to commit to consuming junk food, which has an immediate pleasure-return, than to exercise, which has a more delayed and less pronounced pleasure-return. Commitment to a thin fit body is much more long-term, and requires much more persistence. For those whose bodies signal their status, long-term investment in it is a must, while for those whose bodies are socially neutral or marginalized (the poor especially) pizza may win the day over the gym.

A 'Common Sense' Conclusion

There are many reasons for the steep rise in obesity in the West, many of which are likely to be interactive, some of which might even be contradictory. And despite the almost ubiquitous increases in rates of obesity, being fat has become something of a sin in Western societies, something that the media reflect. An April 2010 *Daily Mail* article about fat children running the risk of being stigmatized reported one father as actually approving stigma 'so that children live a healthy, active life' (Narain, 2010). If during Victorian times, the *orandum est* was that children be seen but not heard, now, *mutatis mutandis*, fat people are not even to be seen – even though lip service is paid to their being 'heard' via reality programmes on television. George Monbiot (2012), in a recent article in *The Guardian*, writes:

> When you raise the subject of over-eating and obesity, you often see people at their worst. The comment threads discussing these issues reveal a legion of bullies who appear to delight in other people's problems. When alcoholism and drug addiction are discussed, the tone tends to be sympathetic. When obesity is discussed, the conversation is dominated by mockery and blame, though the evidence suggests that it may be driven by similar forms of addiction. I suspect that much of this mockery is a coded form of snobbery: the strong association between poor diets and poverty allows people to use this issue as a cipher for something else they want to say, which is less socially acceptable.

The media frame ways of thinking about food and the body: how the former is to be treated and the latter sculpted. In neoliberal societies, both are open to voyeurism and both are commodities for mass visual consumption. Fashion and media did not invent the thinness ideal: it existed in antiquity and has disappeared and re-emerged several times across the centuries. What has changed in recent times, however, is the mass consumption of images of this ideal. This is often accompanied by the mass consumption of images of elite cuisine, as well as of something more material – fast food. The seeming contradictions in the ways that media handle food, cooking, fashion, physical activity and the body reveal how deeply embedded media messages are in the market forces that battle over these types of consumption.

Fighting obesity with the careful application of reason – whether through policy measures or public health education – is a grand project that will fail unless common-sense views of obesity and the forces that create it are understood and dissected. In the first of his six Principles of Semiotics, Jack Solomon (1988) urges us to '[a]lways question the "commonsense" view of things, because "commonsense" is really "communal sense"'. At the base, it is important to understand what the 'tribe' thinks of, and why it enjoys all types of consumption, including consuming the very object that fuels its consumption, the media.

References

Barthes, A. (2009). *Mythologies*. London: Vintage.

Baudrillard, J. (2007 [1970]). *The consumer society: Myths and structures*. London: Sage.

Bordo, S. (1993). *Unbearable weight: Feminism, western culture, and the body*. London: University of California Press.

Bourdieu, P. (1977). *Outline of a theory of practice*. Cambridge: Cambridge University Press.

Brownlie, D. & Hewer, P. (2011). '(Re)covering' the spectacular domestic: Culinary cultures, the feminine mundane, and brand Nigella. *Advertising and Society Review, 12(2)*.

Brumberg, J.J. (1988). *Fasting girls: The emergence of anorexia nervosa as a modern disease*. Cambridge, MA: Harvard University Press.

Caballero, B. (2007). The global epidemic of obesity: An overview. *Epidemiological Review, 29(1)*, 1–5.

Dickson Wright, C. (2012). *A history of English food*. London: Random House UK.

Eco, U. (2010). *On beauty: A history of a Western idea*. London: MacLehose Press, Quercus.

Elias, N. (1978). *The civilizing process: The history of manners*. Urizen Books.

Ephron, N. (Dir.) (2010). Special features. Special ingredients: Creating *Julie & Julia*. Columbia Pictures Industries. DVD: Sony Pictures Home Entertainment.

Farringdon, I.S. & Urry, J. (1985). Food and the early history of cultivation. *Ethnobiology, 5(2)*, 143–57.

Ferris, E. (2003). Parallel discourses and appropriate bodies: Media constructions of anorexia and obesity in the cases of Tracey Gold and Carnie Wilson. *Journal of Communication Inquiry, 27(3)*, 256–273.

Guérard, M. (1977). *Cuisine minceur*. London: Macmillan.
Hosking, R. (1996). *A dictionary of Japanese food: Ingredients and culture.* Rutland: Tuttle Publishing.
Magee, R.M. (2007). Food Puritanism and food pornography: The gourmet semimotics of Martha and Nigella. *Americana: The Journal of American Popular Culture 1900 to Present, 6(2)*, 26–38.
Manbiot, G. (2012, September 10). Alzheimer's could be the most catastrophic impact of junk food. *The Guardian.* Retrieved from http:/www.guardian.co.uk/commentisfree/2012/sep/10/alzheimers-junk-food-catastrophic-effect.
Mennel, S. (1986). *All manners of food: Eating and taste in England and France from the Middle Ages to the present.* 2nd edition. Chicago: University of Illinois Press.
Narain, J. (2010, April 12). Council to ban the word 'obesity' – so fat children don't get offended. *Daily Mail.* Retrieved from http://www.dailymail.co.uk/news/article-1265327/Council-ban-word-obesity--fat-children-dont-offended.html.
O'Neill, M. (2003). Food porn. *Columbia Journalism Review, 42(3)*, 28–45.
Offer, A., Pechey, R. & Ulijaszek, S.J. (2010). Obesity under affluence varies by welfare regimes: The effect of fast food, insecurity, and inequality. *Economics and Human Biology*, *8*, 297–308.
Saguy, A. & Gruys, K. (2010). Constructions of overweight and eating disorders. *Social Problems, 57(2)*, 231–250.
Solomon, J. (1988). *The signs of our time: The secret meanings of everyday life.* New York: Harper & Row.
Stewart, M.L. & Janovicek, N. (2001). Slimming the female body? Re-evaluating dress, corsets, and physical culture in France, 1890s–1930s. *Fashion Theory: The Journal of Dance, Body, and Culture, 5(2)*, 173–193.
Teuteberg, H.J. (2007). The birth of the modern consumer age: Food innovation from 1800. In P. Freedman (ed.), *Food: The history of taste* (pp. 233–262). London: Thomas & Uhdson.
Ulijaszek, S. (2012). Socio-economic status, forms of capital and obesity. *Journal of Gastrointestinal Cancer, 43(1)*, 3–7.

Chapter 5

From Abject Eating to Abject Being: Representations of Obesity in 'Supersize vs. Superskinny'

Karin Eli and Anna Lavis

Introduction

Channel 4's reality programme, 'Supersize vs. Superskinny' has a deceptively simple premise: bringing an obese person and an underweight person into a liminal space – the show's so-called 'feeding clinic' – and having them exchange eating habits so that both participants might learn the error of their ways. In so doing, the programme leads its paired obese and underweight participants through the looking glass of reverse embodiment: there, in the 'clinical' spatiality of de-contextualized kitchens and immaculate dining rooms, the meal exchange sees each undergo an intimate sensory experience of the other's foods and eating habits. It is intended that after a few days, this encounter of extremes, mediated by host Dr Christian Jessen, will provide both participants with the education they need to part with their disordered eating practices. Yet, while 'Supersize vs. Superskinny' purportedly extends its alimentary education to both ends of the 'super' scale, the imminent danger of obesity, and its 'costs' to both the individual participant and society as a whole, is at the heart of its visual narrative.

As scholars across disciplines have argued, obesity is highly stigmatized in Euro-American cultures (see Erdman Farrell, 2011; Evans Braziel & LeBesco, 2001; Gilman, 2008), with body fat increasingly discursively framed as no more than a 'corruption of the flesh whose removal [leaves] the body intact and in better shape' (Klein, 2001: 27). In no previous era have rising rates of obesity – of what has been termed 'globesity' (Delpeutch et al., 2009) – received more media coverage or been more debated across academic disciplines and political arenas. Obesity is now framed in alarmist tones as an 'epidemic', carrying the threat of progressively eroding individual and population health, while increasingly burdening the economies of nation states (Boero, 2007).

By analysing episodes from seasons three to six (2010–2013) of 'Supersize vs. Superskinny', this chapter reflects on how the programme both draws on and visually 'parades' these wider cultural imaginings of fat and obesity, whilst using the resonances of alarm and abjection to construct a visual narrative for our viewing pleasure. As a literal meeting space for body weight extremes, 'Supersize vs. Superskinny' provides a visceral education about the perils of becoming obese; this chapter examines how this message is conveyed through the programme's representations of the obese 'journey'. By moving through the series of 'milestones' that underpin the programme's narrative structure, the chapter traces the ritualized transition from the obese participants' initial 'dangerous' pleasure in food, through the externalization and 'othering' of this food, and to the ultimate experience of 'abject being': an encounter with a disabled, morbidly obese American. It is only through the visceral learning and un-learning performed by the 'supersizer' at each of these stages that 'redemption' – taking the form of a 'new future' – may be achieved. Arguing that the programme co-implicates foods and bodies in a visual rhetoric of abjection, which frames obesity as a singular and individual 'danger issuing from within the identity' (Kristeva, 1982: 71), this chapter demonstrates how 'Supersize vs. Superskinny' positions the tacit learning of abjection as central to the prevention and reversal of obesity within the individual and social body.

The Scale Room: Encountering the Other and Othering Obesity

> All over Britain, dietary crimes are being committed. With an increasingly dysfunctional relationship with food at both ends of the scale, we've rounded up 16 of the worst offenders. We've brought them together for the first time to face the harsh reality of what their eating habits have done. ('Supersize vs. Superskinny', series 5, episode 1)

Thus begins the fifth series of UK Channel 4's 'Supersize vs. Superskinny': the camera panning into a room filled with men and women, eight obese, eight underweight, all in nude-coloured underwear, waiting to be weighed. The room's centrepiece – a large weighing scale – intimates the looming mugshot, each 'criminal' to be assigned a profile in pounds and stones. The participants then encounter the 'other' – their polar opposite, the non-me whose meals they will have to consume, and whose essence they will therefore (partially) embody. This 'other' is intended to act as corrective to their own extremes. As the participants are put into these pairs by Dr Christian, size comparisons immediately ensue: arms are placed next to one another, the relative thickness of torsos estimated: 'I'm twice as big as you'. For the audience, this is a particularly powerful visual premise, where opposing spectacles of the body in extremes can be seen together and directly contrasted. Their extraordinariness is made hyperbolic through this act of pairing, which evokes templates of 'enfreakment' (Thomson, 1996a) – the silencing, distancing and stylizing of bodies to be placed on show for the viewing pleasure/horror of others (Thomson, 1996b: 10). This encounter in the scale room thus signifies the moment at which obesity quite literally takes centre stage and the spectacle, and spectacular visualization, of 'fat' in 'Supersize vs. Superskinny' commences. For the scantily-clad participants whose eyes and voices map their own and the other's contours, this moment is narrative-defining; for them it is now that the disciplining of the 'supersized' body begins. In relation to this disciplining, this moment of encounter sets in motion for the audience a narrative in relation to which we find ourselves uncertainly positioned; the viewer is sometimes invited to watch the unfurling of the obese participants' abjection from the comfortable vantage point of a 'laughing chorus' (Bakhtin, 1984: 207), but at other times we look down to find our bodies implicated and entangled, sensing a burgeoning enfreakment (Thomson, 1996a) within our own corporeality.

Thus, although the programme nominally sets out to educate both its 'superskinny' and its 'supersized' participants, it soon becomes apparent that the obese person is at the focus of the show's critical lens; not all 'dietary crimes', it seems, are equally punishable. Lip service is paid to the education of the skinny people: we see them, for example, being lectured on iron deficiency while strolling through galleries of medical photographs depicting bald spots and bleeding gums. But it is the obese body which the programme's narrative template directly evokes as the object of discipline. Only the 'supersized' participants are forced to confront their foods and bodies viscerally and immediately. That it is obesity that embodies the 'absolute otherness' (Fielder, 1996: xiii) of abject being becomes explicit in the programme's fifth season in particular, which is framed through Dr Christian's visits to Evansville, Indiana (branded America's fattest city), and the medical horrors he encounters there. This performance of 'othering' runs through the three milestones of the participants' journey – the food tube, the meal swap and letters from America – where the 'supersized' participants learn to view their bodies, taste their food, and sense their being-in-the-world through their 'superskinny' foil. And key to these milestones is abjection. To 'face the harsh reality of what their eating habits have done', as the voiceover puts it, and to move teleologically from abjection to a redemption borne of sensory discipline, the obese participants must first learn to embody – or, perhaps, recognize their existing embodiment of – disgust.

The Food Tube: Body/Food Transubstantiations

In seasons three and four, the first milestone of abjection, after the encounter in the scale room, is the food tube. Soon after meeting their 'other', the participants, still clad only in underwear, are joined by Dr Christian, who confronts them with the visual reality of what they 'really' eat. This education, based both on the premise that 'seeing is believing' and on the assumption that what participants believe themselves to eat is erroneous, is accomplished by dropping each participant's weekly intake of food into a clear plastic tube. Seemingly out of nowhere, the participants' meals – discursively framed as evidence of 'criminal' intake – are individually 'dumped' so that each can be 'sized up' and commented on separately. The format of this segment emphasizes, once again, the 'supersizer' as central to the programme's narrative. It is always the food tube of the 'superskinny' person that is viewed first, which allows the show to move towards the dramatic climax –

the ultimate enfreakment – of the 'supersizer's' food tube. The spectacular process of what we might term 'abjectification' that this narrative trajectory achieves is enhanced by the deliberate contrasting of each participant's tube with the other. The visual quelching horror of seeing food, drinks and sometimes cigarettes all mushed up together in a plastic tube is undoubtedly there for the viewer when we watch the 'skinny' person's tube fill up. Yet this is attenuated, and very deliberately ranked into a lesser horror, by both the voiceover and the comments of Dr Christian. In Series four, episode one, for example, Dr Christian says of 'supersized' Louise's food tube, as opposed to that of Josh (who only eats dinner four times a week and never eats breakfast or lunch), 'We're only on breakfast and already Louise's tube is level with Josh's entire week of food'. This discursive framing suggests that, whilst there is recognition that Josh does not eat enough, this process of comparison really only works in one direction; the 'supersizer's' food tube is performed as the more shockingly aberrant. Josh, like the other 'superskinnies', is thereby rendered strangely invisible by his food tube, whilst for Louise, and all the other 'supersizers', there is a hypervisibility that echoes wider discursive formations of obesity. Samantha Murray (2005) has explored this 'hypervisibility', demonstrating how body fat is often understood in solely visual terms rather than in relation to complexities of culture, embodiment or subjectivity. This already-ratified cultural hypervisibility not only resonates through, but is also played on by the food tube segment of 'Supersize vs. Superskinny'. Here, we are lulled into an unfeeling amnesia regarding the personhood of the supersized participants standing vulnerably in their underwear contemplating their week of food. This means that here, as it does in wider stigmatizing cultural imaginings, 'the fat body is read as the corporeal presencing of other, presumably more intrinsic, incorporeal qualities or characteristics' (LeBesco & Evans Braziel, 2001: 3). Yet, the food tube goes even further than this: through the food tube, the 'supersizers' are reduced to nothing more than the fat (on their) body. Its hypervisibility precisely renders them, and their personhood, nothing more than a receptacle of spectacularized visibility.

The food tube has been discontinued in season five to be replaced by a segment in which Dr Christian, instead, makes the 'supersized' participant's favourite food, such as pepperoni, curry or chocolate, to demonstrate to the obese participants all the supposedly 'horrifying' ingredients that sneak, unthought-about, into their diets. Aimed at fostering disgust by making these 'horrors' visible, Dr Christian not infrequently uses a cement mixer to make a week's worth of the participants' favourite foodstuff, thereby de-establishing it as food. Although this act of delinking food from edibility is clearly part of the same process of manufacturing disgust that we saw in the food tube, what this new segment has lost is the elision of food and bodies present there; through its hypervisibility, the food tube led the 'supersizers' to, quite literally, have all their insides hanging out.

That food and the body are blurred in many ways throughout 'Supersize vs. Superskinny' is clear; 'supersized', after all, is a term associated with fast food products and such food allusions are not incidental. Conflation of bodies and food (and food that transubstantiates into flesh) is a strong theme of the show: sandwiches are described as 'bulging' with tuna; 'superskinny' Nick's portions – after many shots of his torso and upper arms – are described as 'puny'; and, upon first meeting 'superskinny' Lynsey, 'supersized' Hugh tells her, 'I've had something like you on a plate with chips before, you know' (5, 1). The equating of food fat and body fat is so entrenched in the programme that when Julie and Zoe swap diets in season six, episode three, it is this linkage that leads the central focus of the obese participant's journey to be momentarily suspended. Unprecedentedly, Julie and Zoe are led together around the gallery of photographs of potential future health problems ensuing from their diets. This is because each – in differing quantities – eats a diet high in saturated fat; they are therefore shown, in tandem, the fatty clogging of arteries, which is a visual experience more habitually confined to the 'supersizer'.

Yet nowhere is this conflation of food and body – and its purpose in the production of abjection – more apparent than in relation to the quite literal viscerality of the food tube. The tube functions as a prosthetic stomach – a visible belly, rendered open, 'dissectible' and perhaps, grotesquely unfinished (Bakhtin, 1984), by our viewing gaze. The belly, described by Ana Carden-Coyne and Christopher Forth (2005: 1) in their work on fat as 'the primary site of incorporation, where food is directly assimilated into the body, where it is literally made into flesh' is visually prominent in the show; there are many shots that focus on the flesh of the abdomen overhanging underwear or striped with stretch marks, in the tradition of what Charlotte Cooper has dubbed 'headless fatties'. As Cooper (2007) says: 'the body becomes symbolic: we are there but we have no voice, not even a mouth in a head, no brain, no thoughts or opinions. Instead we are reduced and dehumanized as symbols of cultural fear: the body, the belly, the arse, food'. Through the corporeal sploshing of the food that comes, with some speed, down the tube's clear plastic insides, the body of the 'supersizer' is turned inside out to render them nothing but belly. Here, in contrast to Bakhtin's (1984, 1998) carnivalesque 'world turned inside out' whereby the fool could become the king, albeit it only for a day, the belly turned inside out renders the 'supersized' person morally abject. Moreover, that there is a carnivalesque order to this process of what we might term moral enfreakment is demonstrated by the fact that this very travesty of the reversal of insides and outsides (re-)establishes and solidifies the moral order of the 'error' of obesity (see Bakhtin, 1984). By making the partially-digested food in the tube stand for the body, and enacting a transubstantiation of food into bodies and bodies into food, the food tube segment implies that the body is unknowable until we see the food that each participant eats. Through this food the obese person becomes 'fat' – their supersizededness is made material whilst also reducing their embodiment to quantifiable (weighed and measured, de-relational, and anti-sensory) consumption. All that is evoked is abjection, rather than any sense of how the participants themselves might feel when they eat.

This moment of 'becoming fat' that is enacted by the food tube's literalizing of the size of the obese person is a significant stage in the journey. The food tube shows us an excess that can hardly – and yet must – be contained. Susan Bordo (2003) describes how cultural imaginings of fat see larger bodies as 'taking up space' – space, perhaps, that is taken from others – which, together with an assumption that fat people eat 'too much' food, aligns fat with greed (a connotation that been pointed out by many scholars, including Sander Gilman [2008]). Fat, thus, is framed as selfish; it signifies an expansion beyond one's socially-allotted limits. 'Supersize vs. Superskinny' employs this framing to place the participants' bodies and personhood into a narrative of constructed projected hubris. Although the participants themselves actually exhibit a deep vulnerability and humility standing in their underwear beside their week's food, the programme frames the supersized participants as having, quite literally, become too big for their boots; too much food in the tube comes to stand not only for too much body, but also for too much personhood, all of which must be contained. To counteract this hubris, 'Supersize vs. Superskinny' sets in motion the production of abjection that aims to cut the obese participants down to size. The burgeoning visual aesthetics of cruelty continues to grow as the programme's narrative moves onto the next milestone of the obese journey, the meal swap.

The Meal Swap: Sensory (Un-)Learning

The meal swap, the centrepiece of the programme, is the site where abjection is enacted and made visual through the sensory experience of the 'superskinny' person. Sitting across from their 'other' as s/he eats, with the 'skinny' person often contorting her/his face, commenting on feeling full, and ending the meal mid-course, the obese participants are imbued with a sense of what their food (should) feel(s) like.

The sensory education offered by 'Supersize vs. Superskinny' does not focus on teaching the fat participants to sense food differently (or enjoy it), but rather on teaching them to feel hunger pangs. Dr Christian frequently mentions hunger sensation as a positive outcome – 'you felt hunger pangs for the first time in years!' – and to take pleasure in that absence (or pain). There is a sense in many episodes that the 'supersized' participants have previously had 'too much' of a relationship with food. Pleasure in food, then, is dangerous. And there is no interest in exploring how the 'supersizers' experience food – only in how they should sense it. We are treated, though, to images of 'skinny' people struggling mightily against the abjection of food – their sensory worlds are delineated all too clearly. Perhaps the audience's embodied identification with fat people in eating would be dangerous as well?

As we have already seen, throughout the show, the boundaries of harm are set in particular ways, with the 'superskinny' person as a mere foil to the 'supersized' person. As such, it is only in relation to the 'supersized' people that eating is represented as problematic during the meal swap. They are the ones who have dysfunctional relationships with food that need sorting out. The thin participants are seen, simply – or simplistically – as not eating enough. So, when Elaine (5, 1) says that she is put off eating by particular colours of food and Marie (5, 8) expresses horror at eating any fat at all and weighs all her food, we are not led to draw any conclusions about their (lack of) engagement with food. The intricacies are left out – all that remains, again, is a focus on amounts. Josh (4, 1), for example, says that 'If I could get away with not eating, I probably would' and the reality of this becomes apparent after he and Louise swap diets and she, subjected to his normal diet, does not eat for 48 hours on days two and three. The unhealthiness – the harm – of this extreme lack of food is glossed over. Dr Christian, instead, talks about Josh's smoking and confronts him with images of the health consequences of tobacco use, not starvation.

In season six, episode five, it is clear that both Hannah and Victoria have emotional relationships with food – that eating and not eating are enmeshed with past experiences and affects. Yet, it is only Hannah's 'overeating' that is represented in this way, and she is even described in the tagline to the episode as a 'teenage comfort eater'. As such, the show employs two very different paradigms of eating – that which can be calculated and weighed, which is de-relational, and that which is more entangled with emotions and selfhood; these share the visual space of the programme, even producing the visuality of the other for our viewing, but they do not, to borrow from Annmarie Mol (2002), 'hang together' neatly. The abject is presented as visual and sensory fact, an accompaniment to the 'hard' data of BMI, cholesterol, blood pressure, calories, fat, and general measures of morbidity. The 'skinny' people are our eyes – or even, our bodies. We are invited to sense through them and to perceive through them. Their horror at the amount of food that they must 'get through' is our embodied horror.

And for the 'supersized' participants, too, their 'superskinny' counterparts become the eyes through which to examine their own reflections. For it is not only in their co-participants that the 'supersizers' encounter the 'other' – through the show, they learn to encounter the 'other' in themselves. As Gail Weiss writes:

> For Kristeva, that which is "lost" or which resists incorporation into the body image is also precisely what makes the coherent body image possible because it marks the boundary between the body image and what it is not. There is a permanent danger that this boundary will be dissolved, however, since the boundary is only reinforced on one side, the Symbolic side. The "other side" is the unnameable, abject domain that continually threatens to overrun its carefully established borders. The fragility of the border in turn undermines the stability and coherence of the body image; as Kristeva notes: "The more or less beautiful image in which I behold or recognize myself rests upon an abjection that sunders it as soon as repression, the constant watchman, is relaxed". (Weiss, 1999: 42)

The obese participants come into the realization of their own abjection – an abjection they were not aware of, an abjection that inheres in their physicality and food. This new-found sense of abjection leads to a profound unsettling of the body image they had heretofore had: of the body they thought they knew.

Letters from America: Future American Selves

As we have seen thus far, 'Supersize vs. Superskinny' argues that the 'supersized' participants don't *see* or *feel* the folly of their ways. They are thus taught to sense their eating as abject through watching their meals drop into the food tube, and observing a clearly disgusted skinny person sitting across from them, struggling not to vomit their food. But, importantly, they are taught to sense their bodies too as abject through being confronted with their American 'future selves' in the Letters from America segment. Critical in the programme's template – and even more to its development in its latest seasons – this section confronts the 'supersized' person with the story of a morbidly obese, often disabled American, whose life story contains some parallels with that of the 'supersized' participant. In later series, this segment has expanded, with the 'supersizers' sent to meet the American participants and, thereby, convene with the people they might become. This pairing of British 'supersizer' and American participant is the ultimate act of 'othering', with the literalization of the abject other as a foreigner. Significantly, there is no equivalent for the 'superskinny' person. This 'other' pairing of the 'supersizer' and the American participant is therefore layered over the already-existing one of the 'supersizer' and 'superskinny', which serves to transfer the 'skinny' participants further into the background, marginalizing their role in the programme as foil further still.

The American participants are often introduced to us as 'headless fatties' (Cooper, 2007), as the camera repeatedly focuses on those body parts most likely to induce abjection. For example, in series 3, episode 6, the first glimpse that the viewer gets of Stephen is a close up shot of his bum. Here, as Colls writes, fat is 'ambiguous; placed simultaneously under the skin yet materialised as a substance in and of itself' (2007: 358). It is fat, not Stephen, that we are looking at here. Once again in 'Supersize vs. Superskinny', personhood and fat are placed in a relationship of inverse correlation. Fat is placed centre stage as the American participants become nothing but their visual obesity. American participants like Stephen are portrayed as ticking clocks of abjection and 'otherness', whose collections of breathing implements and hypertension pills are complemented by technologies of disability, all woven together in sensorily-evocative discourses of abject being (rashes, body odour, fungal infections) and images of humiliating disfigurement (open sores, washing under flaps of skin, being helped to dress). It is also most specifically through this segment that the show closely ties abjection and illness, which allows the full 'morality' – or, rather, moral agenda – of Dr Christian's mission to fight obesity in society as well as in the supersized participant to unfurl. Likewise, the 'supersized' participants are never subjected to comments on their appearance, but they are bombarded with images and discourses of illness, disability, and abjection throughout their stay both in the US and in the feeding clinic.

Following Stephen's 'video letter', British 'supersizer' Allison tells Dr Christian, 'like you said, I'm just the same as him', to which Dr Christian replies, 'it is the same isn't it? And you are teetering on the edge'. By drawing – or, rather, being encouraged to draw – this parallel, Allison forfeits her identity to 'fat' and places herself at the hands of the medical profession in the guise of Dr Christian. Through this pairing, she, like the other British 'supersizers', is portrayed as 'stuck' and in need of help. They are not yet proper moral beings, and are headed only for their future (abject) American selves, in a way that echoes the dynamics of the food tube segment and, therefore, produces a narrative linkage between the American participant and the food tube. That both are seen simply as 'food filled' is not infrequently emphasized by the trips taken around the American participants' kitchens by Dr Christian, who points at often large quantities of unhealthy food whilst chastising the American and talking to the camera. While this televised rebuke is framed as done for the obese participants' 'own good', it envinces an aesthetics of cruelty. As Nietzsche writes, 'to see somebody suffer is nice, to make somebody suffer even nicer' (1994: 46).

Thus, in the letters from America segment, boundaries between continents, bodies, foods, and temporalities are all collapsed into a 'rationalised singularity of obesity' (Throsby, 2012: 1), to borrow from Karen Throsby's discussion of bariatric surgery. This enactment of singularity leaves outside its parameters any 'messy' recognitions of the part played by society in the production and day-to-day living of bodies, and thereby places 'blame' solely within the 'supersized' person and the individual particularities of eating practices. Such rendering of obesity as a singular object is, once again, part of the enfreakment enacted by 'Supersize vs. Superskinny': central to processes of enfreakment is the collapsing of difference into 'a single amorphous category of corporeal otherness' (Thomson, 1996b: 10). Yet, there is a further boundary that is ruptured – the boundary between the obesity on screen and the obesity which may be harboured by our own viewing bodies. Ultimately there are not just two pairings ('supersizer' vs. 'superskinny', and 'supersizer' vs. 'future American self') but three – we are the invisible person in the feeding clinic; we are the unseen obese other whose soon-to-be-dead self will not fit into a normal-sized coffin in Evansville, Indiana and McAllen, Texas. Dr Christian is asking us to look at ourselves, often quite explicitly. So we, too, are abject and must undergo the same processes of learning and un-learning to achieve redemption.

Implications: Abjection as Affective Education

'Supersize vs. Superskinny' ultimately creates life trajectories for its participants, imagined journeys ending either in the horror of the future American self or in the hope of redemption served up by Dr Christian (should they, of course, follow his medically-validated prescriptions for a 'healthy' life). Their potential futures thus played out, it becomes clear what the right (and only) choice is. The moral personhood offered, and indeed opened up, by the show, is not only the individual's responsibility to adopt, but is also a societal imperative. Thus conforming, the 'supersizer' is given an escape route: from turning one's own (quite literal) burden of obesity into a public burden, to becoming a full participant in the moral economy of responsibilized consumption.

With 'Supersize vs. Superskinny' as a self-styled commercial messenger of health education, the participants are portrayed as free-willed, if stubbornly irrational, individuals who make 'bad choices'. To change, they must be confronted not merely with information (which everyone presumably already knows) – but with a sensory education: they need to learn to experience (or acknowledge the already-existent, but stubbornly unrecognized sense of) their bodies as burdensome. Abjection, in this framing, becomes a catalyst to individual responsibility – or, to quote Thaler and Sunstein (2008), an affective 'nudge'.

On the societal level, obesity is constructed as a problem to be prevented and curbed primarily through health education. The success of health education efforts, of course, depends on the receptivity of 'responsible' citizens, ready to develop the 'informed', idealized middle-class habitus which public health education both addresses and constructs. Receptivity, in turn, depends on what we would like to term *sensory consensus*: just as some professionals 'learn to see' to become specialized in certain disciplines (e.g., medicine, anatomy, visual arts), so do citizens 'learn to feel' to become responsible individuals. As Julie Guthman (2011) argues, messages on 'healthy eating' (such as those promulgated by Michael Pollan) are replete with assumptions about taste, body image, and health. These assumptions represent middle class ideals, and as such are meaningful only to a segment of (in that case, US) society; working class and minority citizens, therefore, are to be educated/habituated into idealizing a certain body image (or sense of the body, to be more precise), in order to comply with 'healthy' dietary practices.

In 'Supersize vs. Superskinny', the sensory education of 'supersized' people takes them on a journey through abjection to a socially appropriate moral personhood. This journey, though portrayed as personal, is imbued with the economic – and perhaps moral – cost of obesity, denoted always as a 'disease'. This goes hand in hand with the show's recurrent theme: discursively moving away from structural impacts on the individual consumer, and toward the impact of the obese individual on structural elements, a dynamic made explicit in the show's fifth season, where Dr Christian's adventures in Evansville, Indiana are often contextualized with details on the costs of obesity to the UK National Health Service.

As each 50-minute televised 'supersized' journey draws to a close, the same conclusion – the inescapable image of what constitutes public health burdens – is consistently drawn. Kelly Brownell (1991) suggests that, when neoliberal self-control is prised with health as its emblem, illness becomes a morally abject condition. And as Louise Townend (2009) argues, this moral abjection is tightly linked to poverty – such that obesity, at the crossroad of poverty and illness, is positioned as a moral failing. 'Supersize vs. Superskinny's' sometimes-explicit co-construction of obesity, illness, working-classness, and immorality continuously underlies and informs the discursive and visceral narratives of the show. For the 'supersized' people, then, the 'abjectification' of food and fat connotes a greater moral 'abjectification' of the self.

References

Bakhtin, M. (1984). *Rabelais and his world.* Bloomington: Indiana University Press.
Bakhtin, M. (1998). Carnival and the carnivalesque. In J. Storey (ed.), *Cultural theory and popular culture: A reader* (pp. 250–259). Essex: Prentice Hall.
Boero, N. (2007). All the news that's fat to print: The American 'obesity epidemic' and the media. *Qualitative Sociology, 30*, 41–60.
Bordo, S. (2003). *Unbearable weight: Feminism, Western culture, and the body.* Berkeley and London: University of California Press.
Brownell, K.D. (1991). Personal responsibility and control over our bodies: When expectation exceeds reality. *Health Psychology, 10*, 303–310.
Carden-Coyne, A. & Forth, C. (2005). The belly and beyond: Body, self, and culture in ancient and modern times. In C.E. Forth & A. Carden-Coyne (eds), *Cultures of the abdomen: Diet, digestion and fat in the modern world* (pp. 1–12). New York: Palgrave Macmillan.
Colls, R. (2007). Materialising bodily matter: Intra-action and the embodiment of 'Fat'. *Geoforum, 38*, 353–365.
Cooper, C. (2007). *Headless fatties* [online]. Retrieved from http://www.charlottecooper.net/docs/fat/headless_fatties.htm [accessed February 11, 2012].
Delpeuch, F., Maire, B., Monnier, E. & Holdsworth, M. (2009). *Globesity: A planet out of control?* London: Earthscan.
Erdman Farrell, A. (2011). *Fat shame: Stigma and the fat body in American culture.* New York and London: New York University Press.
Evans Braziel, J. & LeBesco, K. (2001). *Bodies out of bounds: Fatness and transgression.* Berkeley and London: University of California Press.
Fielder, L.A. (1996). Foreword. In R. Garland Thomson (ed.), *Freakery: Cultural spectacles of the extraordinary body* (pp. xiii–xvi). New York: New York University Press.
Gilman, S.L. (2008). *Fat: A cultural history of obesity.* Cambridge: Polity Press.
Guthman, J. (2011). *Weighing in: Obesity, food justice, and the limits of capitalism.* Berkeley and London: University of California Press.
Klein, R. (2001). Fat beauty. In J.E. Braziel & K. LeBesco (eds), *Bodies out of bounds: Fatness and transgression* (pp. 19–38). Berkeley and London: University of California Press.
Kristeva, J. (1982). *Powers of horror: An essay on abjection.* New York: Columbia University Press.
LeBesco, K. (2004). *Revolting bodies: The struggle to redefine fat identity.* Boston: University of Massachusetts Press.

LeBesco, K. & Evans Braziel, J. (2001). Editors' introduction. In J.E. Braziel & K. LeBesco (eds), *Bodies out of bounds: Fatness and transgression* (pp. 19–38). Berkeley and London: University of California Press.

Mol, A. (2002). *The body multiple: Ontology in medical practice.* Duke University Press.

Murray, S. (2005). (Un/be)coming out? Rethinking fat politics. *Social Semiotics, 15*, 153–163.

Nietzsche, F. (1994). *On the genealogy of morality.* Edited by Keith Ansell-Pearson. Cambridge: Cambridge University Press.

Thaler, R.H. & Sunstein, C.R. (2008). *Nudge: Improving decisions about health, wealth, and happiness.* New Haven: Yale University Press.

Throsby, K. (2012). Obesity surgery and the management of excess: Exploring the body multiple. *Sociology of Health and Illness, 34*, 1–15.

Thomson, R.G. (1996a). *Freakery: Cultural spectacles of the extraordinary body.* New York: New York University Press.

Thomson, R.G. (1996b). Introduction: From wonder to error – a genealogy of freak discourse in modernity. In R. Garland Thomson (ed.), *Freakery: Cultural spectacles of the extraordinary body* (pp. 1–19). New York: New York University Press.

Townend, L. (2009). The moralizing of obesity: A new name for an old sin? *Critical Social Policy, 29*, 171–190.

Weiss, G. (1999). The abject borders of the body image. In G. Weiss & H.F. Haber (eds), *Perspectives on embodiment: The intersections of nature and culture* (pp. 41–60). London: Routledge.

PART II
Representations of Science and Policy

In this section, the analytic lens turns to news media reports on scientific research and public health policy concerning obesity and eating disorders. Asking which research findings are selected for reporting, who reports them, and how these findings are represented in different news media, the chapters comprising this section analyse news reports as amalgams of facts, public opinion, institutional and political agendas, and circuitous research dissemination routes. Opening this section is Megan Warin, Tanya Zivkovic, Vivienne Moore and Michael Davies' analysis of media representations of the fetal origins hypothesis as applied to obesity. As the authors demonstrate, while these representations may purport to explain a complex scientific concept, in practice, they employ a reductionist, classed and gendered framing, whereby women (and particularly those living in poverty) are portrayed as the causal agents in transmitting obesity. The use of reductionist media framings to describe complexity is also implicated in Emily Shepherd and Clive Seale's comparative analysis of UK and US media coverage of eating disorders, where the authors find that, while media reports on eating disorders are variable, simplified entertainment-centred framings tend to undergird them. In a similar vein, Abigail Saguy and Rene Almeling find that reductionist framings of blame and alarm colour media reports on medical research concerning obesity. They suggest, moreover, that the media may actively choose to report on those research findings that best fit an alarmist frame. Turning to media coverage of UK obesity policy reports, Stanley Ulijaszek finds that reductionist framings are also applied when media report on public health policies, arguing that media sources rehearse pre-set parameters for evaluating obesity, regardless of the complexity of the policy report at hand. And, closing the section with a systematic analysis of obesity coverage in leading US media sources, Helene Shugart suggests that while multiple popular framings of obesity exist, none is compatible with the discourses employed in public health efforts. Media framings, then, may have substantial implications for the effectiveness of public health policies.

Chapter 6

Mothers as Smoking Guns: Fetal Overnutrition and the Reproduction of Obesity[1]

Megan Warin, Tanya Zivkovic,
Vivienne Moore and Michael Davies

Introduction

In March 2009, an article in the daily State newspaper of South Australia (*The Advertiser*) featured a large photograph of a smiling mother and her new-born baby, warning that 'health problems are passed on through generations' (Stewart, 2009). The headline to the story – 'Mothers' smoking gun' – referred to a cohort study conducted by researchers at the University of Adelaide (including two authors of this chapter) which explicitly states that overweight, pregnant women are more likely to have children, even grandchildren, who are overweight. A similar news item in Australia's national circulation paper (*The Australian*) in the previous month claimed that 'obese women are more likely to have children with a range of birth defects' (Taor, 2009). The warnings are clear – obesity in pregnancy is potentially damaging and it is mothers who are held responsible for their children's ill health.

The media conflation of women's reproductive bodies with smoking guns reflects recent paradigmatic developments in scientific research about the origins of health and disease, and how adult chronic disease might be determined by the 'womb environment'. This new paradigm, termed Barker's hypothesis (or the fetal origins hypothesis), has led to maternal obesity now being understood to contribute to obesity in children through intra-uterine factors that alter fetal metabolism regarding growth, fat deposition, and insulin regulation (Oken & Gillman, 2003). As a result, the interiority of women's reproductive bodies is brought sharply into the media limelight not only as a causal agent in the obesity 'epidemic', but also as the (potential) solution.

We critically examine how the fetal origins hypothesis is reported in popular print media, arguing that reproduction (and more specifically women's reproduction) is

1 Reprinted from: Warin, M., Zivkovic, T., Moore, V. & Davies, M. (2012). Mothers as smoking guns: Fetal overnutrition and the reproduction of obesity. *Feminism & Psychology*, *22(3)*, 360–375.

now a key discursive site in which intergenerational cycles of obesity are being culturally produced and reproduced. To provide evidence of these new discourses in which the bodies of obese, pregnant women are being implicated we examined the reporting of scientific research in Australian print media. In addition to mothers being held legally and morally culpable for overfeeding and neglect of fat children, we found that the reporting of scientific research compounds blame by suggesting that women are responsible for 'programming' their baby for a lifetime of obesity. A new and powerful meta-discourse has emerged in which women are blamed for *both* their reproductive physiology and their social role as mothers, thus constructing women as potentially contaminating future generations by creating obesity lineages.

Of course this discourse of blame did not appear out of thin air; blaming the bodies and behaviours of pregnant women for misshapen fetuses lingers on from our historical understandings of disease causation. Mother blame is not a new phenomenon and historians (Ladd-Taylor & Umansky, 1998) and feminist scholars (Litt, 2000; Singh, 2004) have noted how women have long been accused of smothering children and causing all manner of 'ills' such as homosexuality, schizophrenia, autism and anorexia to name a few. While the concept of mother blame has 'extraordinary elasticity' (Blum, 2007: 203), we argue that the shifting historical discourses of maternal appetites, the scientific location of obesity through the fetal origins of disease, and the popularization of this 'new science' now provide a singular space for the overweight, maternal body to take centre stage. Fat, pregnant bodies are constructed as bio-cultural anxieties, distilling biological and social causes into the one embodied location. Coupled with a neoliberal agenda that emphasizes self-governance and individual responsibility, this powerful meta-discourse (Nerlich, 2009) provides a compelling web of individual and gendered blame for the obesity 'epidemic'.

The Obese, Pregnant Body

Demi Moore's infamous *Vanity Fair* cover in 1991 was a sensational prelude to the idea that good mothers are closely aligned with the ideal neoliberal citizen. Since her cover, photos and stories of pregnant and post-partum celebrities have proliferated in various popular media. Although the consumption of celebrity pregnancies (Danni Minogue, Britney Spears, Angelina Jolie, Heidi Klum and Nicole Richie) – with their neat bumps, well supported breasts, glowing skin, and radiantly energized appearance – communicates a distorted image of expectant mothers and emphasizes the social controls that ordinarily discipline mother's bodies, a fetishization of pregnant celebrities (and 'yummy mummies') has helped to shape new standards of bodily deportment and appearance toward which the pregnant woman is expected to aspire. Foucauldian issues of surveillance and pregnancy policing have been well documented in feminist literature (cf. Ussher, 2006; Longhurst, 2008; Fox, Nicolson & Heffernan, 2009), and the price of mothers-to-be not complying with the dominant ideals of 'good motherhood' are high. Women who don't self-regulate or ignore dominant pregnancy practices are especially beholden to public scathing, as they present what Skeggs (2005: 968) calls a 'constitutive limit to propriety' within both celebrity culture and wider social life.

Once considered healthy, the storage of fat was an acceptable and 'natural' part of pregnancy. Indeed, pregnancy, as understood in recent 'western' history, was a period in which a woman could, albeit temporarily, guiltlessly gain weight; 'eat for two' and rest from exercise. In recent times, however, anxieties about the spread of the 'obesity epidemic' has led fat to be demonized and pathologized as a disease (cf. Campos et al., 2005; Orbach, 2006; Murray, 2008; Moffat, 2010), no matter *which* body it appears on. In a climate where obesity has become a potent signifier for neglect of self (and others), pregnant women are no longer encouraged to eat for two (Bell et al., 2009; Keenan & Stapleton, 2010: 371), and a new regime of dietary practices and recommended weights for mothers-to-be and pregnant women has been promoted by clinical, public health and biomedical experts.

Good mothering practices now begin *before* conception (Lupton, 1996; Fox, 2009), and preconception care is promoted as 'the most loving and responsible choice you and your partner can make together, not only for you and your child's health, but also for future generations' (McDowell, 2005, cited in Possamai-Inesedy, 2006). Obese, even overweight, mothers-to-be should exercise and lower their calorie intake in order to reduce their Body Mass Index (BMI). Additionally, and like all women, they are expected to ensure the optimal conditions for fertility by avoiding substances such as caffeine, alcohol and nicotine, and supplementing their diets with folic acid and other vitamins and minerals. Vigilant attention to their dietary requirements should continue throughout pregnancy, with a regular intake of folic acid in the first trimester and scheduled blood tests to detect nutritional deficiencies at routine intervals. Still abstaining from alcohol and other toxins and consuming a well-balanced diet, the mother should ideally breastfeed, then, when her baby is eventually weaned, nutritious meals should be prepared. Effectively, the 'good mother', responds to a discourse that requires her to act responsibly (Goodwin & Huppatz, 2010: 5), and perform labour-intensive (Hays, 1996) food preparation practices to avoid any potential risks and nourish the body of her child.

'Biological Postcards': The Popularization of Barker's Hypothesis

These disciplinary regimes reflect not only an obsession with the management of 'healthy' bodies, but are now linking 'pre-pregnancy appropriate weight, weight gain and nutrition in pregnancy with satisfactory fetal outcomes and increasingly, with infant health over the life-course' (Keenan & Stapleton, 2010: 371). This new attention to the fetus not only reflects a concern for fetal personhood (Ruddick, 2007) but is supported by scientific developments in the early origins of disease that trace chronic disease in adults back to the intra-uterine environment.

From the late 1980s, research conducted by UK physician and epidemiologist David Barker and his colleagues advanced the theory that chronic disease originated, at least in part, in early life. Barker and his colleagues' work (1986; 1990) led to a profound paradigmatic shift in medical understanding and knowledge, as low birth weight and intra-uterine growth retardation (caused by under-nutrition during fetal development) are presented as important indicators or signals of an elevated risk for many adult diseases (cf. Moore & Davies, 2008). In other words, many chronic adult diseases (especially diabetes and heart disease) are seen as having origins in the intra-uterine environment or early infancy (as well as being influenced by later environmental and life style factors). Throughout the 1990s, evidence of associations (statistical connections) between low birth weight and increased risk of chronic disease in adulthood accumulated. In 1995 the *British Medical Journal* named this 'discovery' the 'Barker Hypothesis', an expression that Barker rejected in favour of 'the fetal origins hypothesis' (Warin et al., 2011). In the science community this new insight became the focus of a major international research effort, and in 2010 *Time Magazine* called Barker's hypothesis a 'pioneering New Science' that turned 'pregnancy into a scientific frontier' (Paul, 2010).

Although the main focus of the field now known as 'developmental origins of adult health and disease' has been on the effects of poor fetal nutrition and low birth weight, the issue of maternal and hence fetal overnutrition is of growing importance in the context of the current global obesity 'epidemic' (McMillen et al., 2008). By the early 2000s, the fetal origins hypothesis had become part of the child obesity lexicon, extending the understanding of obesity 'back to the future', and locating the origins and potentiality of obesity in the fetal environment.

Ebbeling and colleagues (2002: 475), in a landmark paper on the childhood obesity 'crisis', reported an:

> intriguing hypothesis that prenatal overnutrition might affect lifelong risk of obesity. According to this hypothesis, maternal obesity increases transfer of nutrients across the placenta, inducing permanent changes in appetite, neuroendocrine functioning, or energy metabolism … The implications of these findings are formidable: the obesity epidemic could accelerate through successive generations independent of further genetic or environmental factors.

The simplified 'truth' of the maternal origins hypothesis is that weight gain during pregnancy (or maternal obesity pre-pregnancy) can lead to fetal overnutrition, high birth-weight and contribute to childhood obesity independent of the family circumstance (La Coursiere et al., 2005).

Although many researchers investigating fetal origins in the scientific community speak of epidemiological uncertainty, caution and degrees of imprecision (Susser and Levin, 1999; Moore & Davies, 2008; Wells, 2010: 291), the media reporting of these 'new scientific findings' follows a simple storyline, and suggests that as women become too large, their fetuses also grow too large, and as a result 'obesity is programmed in the womb' (*The Times*, 2010). It is now frequently reported that: 'women who are overweight or obese are 2 to 2.5 times more likely to have heavier babies ... and larger babies create problems with delivery, and are more at risk of infection, diabetes, obesity and heart disease in later life' (Shepherd, 2009). 'Obese mums-to-be [are thus] urged to diet' (Hall and Davis, 2009), as 'the first nine months [can shape] the rest of your life' (Paul, 2010). A reductive account of the fetal origins of disease is gold for scientific journalists, for obesity is both individualized and gendered, and characterized in the popular press as 'a mother of a problem' (Parker, 2009: 1).

A number of scholars have examined the media reporting of new scientific research and 'have found that this type of media tends to lack critical coverage or comment by journalists ... [and neglects] both the tentative nature of scientific inquiry and its political context' (Parker, 2000: 4; Dyck, 1995). In spite of this, 'scientific journalism' relies on authoritative discourse, and locates its reporting in a context where 'scientific knowledge continues to hold cultural authority as objective, rational and empirical' (Parker, 2009: 2). Through this powerful legitimization, scientific journalism becomes simultaneously a crucial source of scientific and public health information (Petersen et al., 2009; Boero, 2007; Saguy and Almeling, 2008), and 'a key contributor to the shaping and definition of public health issues as social problems' (Maher et al., 2010: 236). In relation to obesity, Monaghan et al. (2010) describe the media as 'amplifiers/moralizers' as they sensationalize, stereotype and repeatedly focus on 'dramatic' or 'moralizing' aspects of obesity.

Our Study

In 2009 we examined the reporting of obesity over a three-month period (1 January to 31 March 2009) in three metropolitan Australian newspapers – *The Advertiser*, *The Australian* and *The Sydney Morning Herald. The Sydney Morning Herald*, owned by Fairfax Media, and *The Australian* of News Limited, are both broadsheets. *The Australian*, the only national newspaper, has a broader nationwide audience than *The Sydney Morning Herald*, one of the main newspapers published in Sydney. Owned by Murdoch's News Corporation, *The Advertiser* is a tabloid-format newspaper and has the widest circulation in Adelaide. These three newspapers were selected to represent Australia's two dominant media outlets (Fairfax and Murdoch) and different readership and circulation. In order to collect data on visual images we opted against using text-based databases such as Factiva or LexisNexis and manually searched microfilm of the newspapers in our sample. We sourced 181 articles that included at least two of our search terms (obesity/obese AND pregnancy, parenting, child, eating and diet), made multiple copies of each original (to allow for multiple analysis), and conducted a thematic analysis of text and visual images (cf. Bernard, 2010). This involved identifying and describing both implicit and explicit themes within the data and critically exploring the relationships between these themes (for example, the recurrent links between childhood obesity and mothering). We also compared our results with two other Australian studies on media representations of maternal responsibility and obesity (Maher et al., 2010; Malik, 2007).

Maternal Blame

In our media sample, obesity was frequently constructed as a parenting issue and was closely aligned with food consumption. When obesity was constructed in terms of parental responsibility, the onus was on the parent to help their child lose weight for the specific purpose of reducing overweight-associated health problems. As we (Zivkovic et al., 2010) and others (Boero, 2009; Maher et al., 2010; McNaughton, 2011) have highlighted, this 'parent' is consistently coded as 'the mother', 'entrenching women's roles as managers of children's health and inequitably blaming them for childhood obesity' (Maher et al., 2010: 236).

As Malik (2007) notes in her discourse analysis of how mothers of overweight and obese children are portrayed in the Australian media, mothers are often singled out as the culprit of childhood obesity, with headlines such as:

> "Fat mums set the trend for obese kids". (Fox, 2005)
>
> "Fat kids? Yes, Mum's the word". (Cornes, 2006)
>
> "A large legacy – Overweight children may not have to look too far to find the reason – it could all be mum's fault". (Steele, 1999)

'Bad' mothers are morally denigrated as overly permissive ('Refrigerator mums') or relying on junk food ('McMums'), and often blamed for an epidemic in childhood obesity because of a perceived lack of education and lack of care for children. Even '30 years of feminist careerism' (Malik, 2007: 13) is used to blame women being time poor, not making 'home cooked' meals and working outside of the home. For example, in January 2010 London buses and billboards were awash with the slogan 'Career women make bad mothers'. Following public outcry (predominately from working mothers) the Outdoor Advertising Association (who ran the ad campaign in an attempt to promote the effectiveness of billboard advertising) removed them. Such reporting effectively uses what Armstrong refers to a 'medical-moral authority' (2003: 189), in that women who fail to act 'maternally' are held morally responsible and culpable for adverse health outcomes in their children.

In contemporary 'western' societies mothers continue to be held culpable for making the wrong choices in regards to their fetuses' wellbeing. Pregnant bodies and the fetuses they contain are increasingly accessible to the medical and legal professions for inspection and intervention (Epstein, 1995: 140). This has resulted in a shift in pregnancy discourses from maternal health to a concern with fetal personhood (Ruddick, 2007). In this new discourse of fetal personhood, mothers can be 'constructed as antagonistic towards their fetus, who becomes an object of collective concern, with its own public identity as the potential [healthy] citizen' (Longhurst, 1999, cited in Fox et al., 2009: 62). Fetuses and children are portrayed as innocent victims in need of protection from irresponsible parents, and in some cases mothers have been prosecuted for neglect and abuse in raising obese children (Zivkovic et al., 2010).

Media headlines amplify this failure of duty of care in terms of women's biological and social roles as mothers. Childhood obesity, it is claimed, 'might start in the womb' (Brown, 2009), and lies in the 'improper' nutrients supplied to fetuses by their mothers. In response to scientific reports in early 2009, Australian broadsheets had stories with headlines such as: 'Obese mums-to-be urged to diet' (Hall and Davis, 2009), 'Weighty problems born of bad diet in pregnancy' (Brown, 2009), 'Overweight mums putting newborns at greater risks' (Shepherd, 2009), 'Breastfed children least likely to be abused by mothers' (Taor, 2009) and 'Child neglect linked to [breast] feeding' (Medew, 2009).

The storyline to these headlines positions women as responsible for obesity and other chronic diseases in their children if they do not prepare their bodies for pregnancy, do not maintain their bodies during pregnancy, do not breast feed, do not put the right choices in lunchboxes or make nutritious, home cooked meals (cf. Fox et al., 2009; Malik, 2007). Levels of responsibility attributed to mothers in relation to obesity occur at key stages of a child's development, travelling from the 'placenta to breast, from breast to lunchbox, from lunchbox to the dinner table' (Malik, 2007: 46). If women do not accept their 'natural' responsibilities as caregivers (both biologically and through social roles) they fall into what Blum (2007) calls a mother-valour/mother-blame binary. Mothers who fail to perform these key maternal activities are held 'responsible for [poor] child outcomes and thus for the health of families, future citizens, and the nation' (Blum, 2007: 202).

The Permeable Womb

Locating the source of high birth-weight and childhood obesity in the generative female body marks a long history of association between women's bodies and that which is considered dangerous. Hailed as a monstrosity, Epstein (1995) and Ussher (2006) note that the female capacity for reproduction was considered an act of horror during the Enlightenment, and well before the scientific classifications of women's bodily parts and functions in the nineteenth century, birth disabilities and malformations were seen to signify the desires and cravings of mothers. According to a widespread belief, it was the passions bound up with maternal appetites that posed the greatest threat to the assumed permeability of pregnant bodies. A pregnant woman's appetite (including the ingestion of foods, drinks and other sensory experiences such as fear and lust) was the explicit mechanism that transferred the effect from maternal environment to fetus (Kukla, 2005: 14). Pregnancy was thus a dangerous process, for women's appetites increased, which in turn increased the possibility of harmful passions and appetites corrupting the fetus.

This historical assigning of responsibility for defective births to mother's minds and bodies is, according to Epstein (1995: 155), indicative of a 'legacy of blaming the mother for her children's appearance and behaviour', and it 'serves to justify a wide range of strategies for containing women's minds by containing women's bodies'. In the eighteenth and nineteenth centuries, these measures included the restraining and hospitalization of women in order to calm their minds, reduce their passions and decrease their chance of having a deformed infant.

While knowledge and practices surrounding pregnancy have significantly changed through time, Kukla (2005) suggests that preoccupations with pregnant bodies and potentiality to harm the fetus still govern our imagination. In the news media, maternal obesity is constructed as harming the fetus, and it is the uncontrollable appetites of mothers to be that are blamed for the obesity epidemic:

> Blame your mother if you're overweight. Sounds Freudian and perhaps a bit mean, but a breakthrough study on obesity indicates that the path to becoming a podgy adult begins in the womb. (*Taranaki Daily News*, July 2007)

Intergenerational Reproduction of Obesity

While several academics have highlighted the discourses of risk associated with such representations of maternal obesity (Keenan & Stapleton, 2010; Maher et al., 2010; McNaughton, 2011), we argue that the focus on intergenerational 'passing on' or transmission of fat from mothers to fetuses and babies constructs women and their reproductive capacities as potentially polluting. In line with social anthropologist Mary Douglas' concept of 'matter out of place' (1966), pregnant bodies are already symbolically marked as dangerous because the flow of reproductive fluids represents a transgression of bodily boundaries. Pregnant bodies expand with fat, fetus and fluid. Corporeal boundaries become confused and blurred 'with the merging of two bodies' (Johnson, 2010: 252) as the fetus distorts the category of subjectivity, feeding from the mother's body through the placenta.

Fat too is 'matter out of place'. In a world of plenty, it represents gluttony, it provokes disgust, contravenes the standards of ideal beauty, and is at the core of our dietary restrictions and understandings of bodily purity (Murray, 2005). The boundary between the body and the world is challenged and reconfigured by fat, which represents an invasion of the body by the world (Huff, 2001: 44). This invasion means that the fat body (which translates to personhood) is discursively constructed as a failed body project, existing as a 'deviant, perverse form of embodiment' (Murray, 2005: 155). Women who are obese and pregnant are thus all the more visible, and doubly grounded in biology (Unnithan-Kumar, 2011: 6) as reproductive, and as fat. Consequently, fat, pregnant women are a threat to the fetus:

> Researchers believe fat mothers pass their obesity to their children. Professor Ross Shepherd, from University of Queensland's Nutrition Research Centre, said initial studies indicated maternal obesity was related to overweight infants. (Steele, 1999: 3)

The contravention of order is not limited to the transgression of external and internal bodily boundaries: dangerous substances also course through the interiority of women's bodies. Bell et al. (2009) argue that in public health discourses on Fetal Alcohol Spectrum Disorder (FASD), smoking when pregnant, and childhood overnutrition, the exposure of a fetus to alcohol, drugs, or fat carries the risk of damaging the child's health. 'Modes of seepage' permeate at the intersection of mother and fetus, a connection between placenta and umbilical cord, where matter can pass from one being to another in a process of feeding and excretion.

However, instead of exploring this placental process as a protective barrier that limits exposure of the fetus to harmful substances, the media (and some social scientists) completely ignore this clinical evidence and revert to a simplistic discourse in which pregnancy and the womb operate as a 'performance of contagion … where the passage of fluid inside the pregnant body, backwards and forwards between the pregnant woman and the fetal entity, enacts the process of contagion' (Maher, 2001: 201). Thus transmission of fat is no longer presented as a *potential* risk: instead intergenerational *certainty* of transmission is presented. Such logic couples appetite and emotions of guilt through successive generations of gendered blame:

> Gulp … You are what your grandmother ate … Research by the Victor Chang Institute shows that what mothers and grandmothers ate during pregnancy affects the health of a particular generation through the genes that are passed on. (*The Sydney Morning Herald*, 2006: 45)

Pregnant Bodies as Smoking Guns

The 'Mothers' smoking gun' (Stewart, 2009) article, cited at the beginning of this chapter, extends the potentiality of harm to the interiority of women's bodies. Despite the lead-researcher (one of the authors of this chapter) emphasizing to the journalist that life course and intergenerational health are 'intertwined in very complex ways' the representation of obese women as 'smoking guns' took precedence. This representation feeds into a simplistic discourse of genetics and deviance; the smoking gun is a popular media metaphor for understanding complex medical relationships where there appears strong circumstantial evidence for a causal relationship between an exposure and a disease process, but where the direct causal mechanism is obscure or unavailable for direct observation. A smoking gun represents a gun that has already 'gone off' and as such presents indisputable evidence of a crime that has been committed. In this case, the crime is to be overweight and pregnant, thus harming the unborn fetus. It is not the microscopic or invisible workings of genes that are the gun, but obese women's bodies in pregnancy that are viewed as culpable.

The metaphor of (fat, pregnant) women as smoking guns is limited and inadequate, as the overnutrition hypothesis speaks to a bodily environment (the womb) that is very much mediated by the socio-economic environment in which the woman is situated. In reducing scientific understandings to genetic determinism, the interplay between bodies and their socio-cultural context is entirely overlooked. Within the fetal overnutrition hypothesis, there is no social circumstance without risk to the mother and the child. Every action involving a diet, food, and social practice is a compromise of interests, hazards, and likelihoods. Every action is constrained by a range of factors, whether social or biological. It is equally inadequate to attempt to explain the body of the mother as entirely reducible to either genetic or intra-individual motivational factors. The body of the mother is therefore a socio-biological accomplishment, the product of selection and survivorship pressures across generations that is in turn shaped by the social context within a lifetime.

The ways in which our bodily environment is mediated by diverse social factors is overlooked in the imagery of the smoking gun and in other print media claims that childhood obesity is *triggered* by 'mothers who eat junk food during pregnancy' (*Science Daily*, 2007), or that fat, pregnant women 'condemn their children to a life of overeating and obesity' (Connolly, 2008). In narrowing the frame of potential risks to the behaviour and biology of expectant women, the bodies of mothers are solely blamed for the misfeeding of their children, even in utero.

In this popularist discourse of the maternal lineage of fat transmission, men are absent from the production and reproduction of obesity across generations. It is assumed that the mother, and only the mother, influences the fetal environment and effects the transmission of obesity in her children. Recent studies, however, contest this position, finding the association between maternal and offspring BMI is comparable to that between paternal and offspring BMI, and concluding that intergenerational obesity involves both the father and the mother (Davey Smith et al., 2007; Kivimäki et al., 2007; Cole et al., 2008; Hawkins et al., 2009). And, among studies which find a stronger correlation between maternal and offspring BMI than that between paternal and offspring BMI, it does not necessarily follow that offspring BMI is an indicator of offspring fat mass during childhood (Lawlor et al., 2008). Lawlor et al. (2008: 491) caution that 'developmental overnutrition related to greater maternal BMI is unlikely to have driven the recent obesity epidemic'.

One interpretation of these data is that while there are specific clinical conditions in pregnancy that can directly influence the growth trajectory of the fetus, and thereby the offspring, these factors can be largely swamped within an environment where the majority of the adult population is overweight or obese. Hence, most of the variation in child BMI may be attributable to social factors common to both the mother and father, and not the direct biological effect of maternally mediated fetal nutrition operating specifically in pregnancy. Again, while the mother may be holding a smoking gun, so too, is the father.

Implications and Conclusion

In this chapter we have shown how women's reproductive bodies are entangled in historical, scientific and media discourses that intimately link the behaviours and biology of mothers with harm to the fetus. The reporting on the 'new science' of the fetal overnutrition hypothesis now extends the gendered nature of infant feeding practices to the interiority (including molecular and genetic levels) of women's bodies. Social environments have segued into intra-uterine environments, in which fat, pregnant mothers can transmit obesity on to their children and future generations. Coupled with a political shift to individual responsibility and moralizing discourses on obesity (Wright & Harwood, 2009), maternal obesity has become a powerful meta-discourse of blame.

Reductive understandings of obesity lead to reductive solutions. Blaming mothers for children's excess weight in both biological and social terms narrows the cause of 'the obesity problem' and therefore the solution to the individual bodies of women. Clinical suggestions of pharmacological contraception, gastrointestinal surgery and the frequent use of weighing stations, all proposed to reduce obesity in women (e.g., Kral, 2004), girls and young women, have proliferated, yet are misplaced. Alarmingly, it is not only the corpulent pregnant woman who is to blame for obesity. Kral (2004: 1544), a US Surgeon writing in the prestigious journal *Paediatrics* in 2004, argues that all women, even 'newborn girls', have the potential to become 'doubly damaging', both polluted and polluting, since fat is passed on through the female body. Accordingly, the only way to curb the obesity epidemic is to 'urgently' target girls and young women: '[f]rom birth to menarche, behaviour modification in mothers and children should be the first choice' in obesity prevention (Kral, 2004: 1544).

While Kral's view is extreme, McNaughton (2011: 1) argues that 'core assumptions at the heart of obesity science have been taken up uncritically in medical arenas focused on conception, pregnancy and reproduction and that this is providing new opportunities for the surveillance, regulation and disciplining of "threatening" (fat) female bodies'. We would agree that the Foucauldian gaze is firmly on the interiority of women's bodies, but we do not take the fetal origins field as a homogenous one. Some scientists working in this field do critique the narrow framing of obesity causality (Warin et al., 2011), arguing that this draws attention away from the very real structural inequalities in health care, education and employment that are often felt hardest by women and minorities (Boero, 2009: 118). As Kukla (2008) notes, public discourse tends to focus on individual responsibility and displays of will-power (or failure of these), rather than the structural conditions that enable or undermine people's ability to make choices over the long term (Kukla, 2008: 83).

Longhurst (1999) noted that pregnancy is a biological process but exists within socio-cultural, economic and political realms and is both spatially and temporally located (cited in Fox et al., 2009: 57). If we focus on the relationships between the social and the biological, and the ways in which they fundamentally interact with each other, then we have a much more powerful framework to understand gendered bodies and the social determinants of health. Barker's work potentially offers a way to reduce social inequalities in health by giving attention to the living conditions, health and nutrition of young women, pregnant mothers and their children. Fetal origins, for example, provides a compelling framework to understand the high rates of obesity amongst women in disadvantaged populations. In a discussion of the obesity amongst the Pima Indians of Arizona, Wells argues that 'obesity arrived [most notably for the Pima women] in combination with poverty and US government rations of sugar and flour' (2010: 296). Poor maternal diets, gender bias through preferential feeding of male children, and fetal exposure to maternal work during pregnancy means that obesity is structurally embedded in socio-cultural contexts. Addressing women's livelihoods will bring particular benefits to their health, whilst further passing these on to subsequent generations.

Our research focuses on the ways in which the politics of mothering and individualized (gendered) responsibility is implicated in obesity debates and policy (Moore & Davies, 2008; Zivkovic et al., 2010). The media are central to this politics as it is part of a neoliberal paradigm that aims to individualize responsibility and individualize the biocultural. In its shallow approach, it reaches into women's bodies to locate obesity as simply a matter of good or bad mothering. Our research aims to invert the gaze to phenomena *outside the body* – to focus on bodily action, biological endowment, evolutionary history and the organization of society (and not just one of these). This approach means challenging the communication of knowledge that is strongly influenced by the media's power to characterize women's bodies (in both their reproductive capacities and social roles) in ways that make it seem 'natural' to blame them for obesity transmission across generations.

References

Armstrong, E. (2003). *Conceiving risk: Bearing responsibility*. Baltimore: The Johns Hopkins University Press.

Barker, D. (1990). The fetal and infant origins of adult disease. *British Medical Journal, 301(6761)*, 1111.

Barker, D. & Osmond, C. (1986). Infant mortality, childhood nutrition, and ischaemic heart disease in England and Wales. *Lancet, 327(8489)*, 1077–1081.

Bell, K., McNaughton, D. & Salmon, A. (2009). Medicine, morality and mothering: Public health discourses on fetal alcohol exposure, smoking around children and childhood overnutrition. *Critical Public Health, 19(2)*, 155–170.

Bernard, H. & Ryan, G. (2010). *Analyzing qualitative data: Systematic approaches*. Thousand Oaks, CA: Sage.

Blum, L. (2007). Mother-blame in the Prozac nation: Raising kids with invisible disabilities. *Gender & Society, 21*, 202–226.

Boero, N. (2007). All the news that's *fat* to print: The American 'Obesity Epidemic' and the media. *Qualitative Sociology, 30(1)*, 41–61.

Boero, N. (2009). Fat kids, working moms, and the 'Epidemic of Obesity'. In Rothblum, E. & Solovay, S. (eds), *The fat studies reader* (pp. 113–119). New York: New York University Press.

Brown, J. (2009). Weight problems born of bad diet in pregnancy. *The Sydney Morning Herald*, 5 February, p. 17.

Campos, P., Saguy, A., Ernsberger, P., et al. (2006). The epidemiology of overweight and obesity: Public health crisis or moral panic? *International Journal of Epidemiology, 35(1)*, 55–60.

Cole, T., Power, C. & Moore, G. (2008). Intergenerational obesity involves both the mother and the father. *American Journal of Clinical Nutrition, 87*, 1535.

Connolly, E. (2008). Mum's diet shapes a child's future weight. *The Sunday Telegraph*, January 27. Retrieved from http://www.news.com.au/features/mums-diet-shapes-a-childs-future-weight/story-e6frfl49-1111115406021.

Cornes, N. (2006). Fat kids? Yes, mum's the word. *Sunday Mail*, 17 September, p. 110.

Davey Smith, G., Steer, C., Leary, S. & Ness, A. (2007). Is there an intra-uterine influence on obesity? Evidence from parent-child associations in the Avon longitudinal study of parents and children (ALSPAC). *Archives of Disease in Childhood, 92*, 876–880.

Douglas, M. (1966). *Purity and danger: An analysis of the concepts of pollution and taboo*. London: Routledge & Kegan Paul.

Dyck, J. (1995). *Manufacturing babies and public consent: Debating the new reproductive technologies*. London: Macmillan.

Ebbeling, C., Pawlak, D. & Ludwig, D. (2002). Childhood obesity: Public-health crisis, common sense cure. *Lancet, 360*, 473–482.

Epstein, J. (1995). The pregnant imagination, fetal rights, and women's bodies: A historical inquiry. *Yale Journal of Law & the Humanities, 7*, 139–162.

Fox, M. (2005). Fat mums set the trend for obese kids. *The Sunday Mail*, 30 January, p. 29.

Fox, R., Nicolson, P. & Heffernan, K. (2009). Pregnancy police? Maternal bodies, surveillance and food. In P. Jackson (ed.), *Changing families, changing food* (pp. 57–74). Basingstoke: Palgrave Macmillan.

Goodwin, S. & Huppatz, K. (eds) (2010). *The good mother: Contemporary motherhoods in Australia*. Sydney: Sydney University Press.

Hall, L. & Davis, K. (2009). Obese mums-to-be urged to diet. *The Sydney Morning Herald*, March 30, p. 3.

Hawkins, S., Cole, T., Law, C. & the Millennium Cohort Study Child Health Group (2009). An ecological systems approach to examining risk factors for early childhood overweight: Findings from the UK Millennium Cohort Study. *Journal of Epidemiology and Community Health*, *63*, 147–155.

Hays, S. (1996). *The cultural contradictions of motherhood*. New Haven: Yale University Press.

Huff, J. (2001). A 'horror of corpulence': Interrogating Bantingism and mid-nineteenth-century fat-phobia. In J. Braziel & K. LeBesco (eds), *Bodies out of bounds: Fatness and transgression* (pp. 39–59). Berkeley: University of California Press.

Johnson, S. (2010). Discursive constructions of the pregnant body: Conforming to or resisting body ideals? *Feminism and Psychology*, *20(2)*, 249–254.

Keenan, J. & Stapleton, H. (2010). Bonny babies? Motherhood and nurturing in the age of obesity. *Health, Risk & Society*, *12(4)*, 369–383.

Kivimäki, M., Lawlor, D., Davey Smith, G., et al. (2007). Substantial intergenerational increases in body mass index are not explained by the fetal overnutrition hypothesis: The Cardiovascular Risk in Young Finns Study. *American Journal of Clinical Nutrition*, *86*, 1509–1514.

Kral, J. (2004). Preventing and Treating Obesity in Girls and Young Women to Curb the Epidemic. *Obesity Research*, *12(10)*, 1539–1546.

Kukla, R. (2005). *Mass hysteria: Medicine, culture and mother's bodies*. Lanham, MD: Rowman & Littlefield.

Kukla, R. (2008). Measuring mothering. *The International Journal of Feminist Approaches to Bioethics*, *1(1)*, 67–90.

La Coursiere, D., Bloebaum, L., Douncan, J. & Varner, M. (2005). Population-based trends and correlates of maternal overweight and obesity, Utah 1991–2001. *American Journal of Obstetrics and Gynecology*, *192(3)*, 832–839.

Ladd-Taylor, M. & Umansky, L. (eds) (1998). *'Bad' mothers*. New York: New York University Press.

Lawlor, D., Timpson, N., Harbord, R., et al. (2008). Exploring the developmental overnutrition hypothesis using parental-offspring associations and FTO as an instrumental variable. *Public Library of Science Medicine*, *5(3)*, 1–10.

Lawrence, R. (2004). Framing obesity: The evolution of news discourse on a public health issue. *The Harvard International Journal of Press/Politics*, *9*, 56–75.

Litt, J. (2000). *Medicalized motherhood*. New Brunswick, NJ: Rutgers University Press.

Longhurst, R. (1999). Pregnant bodies, public scrutiny: 'Giving' advice to pregnant women. In E. Teather (ed.), *Embodied geographies: Spaces, bodies and rites of passage* (pp. 78–90). London: Routledge.

Longhurst, R. (2008). *Maternities: Gender, bodies and space*. New York: Routledge.
Lupton, D. (1996). *Food, the body and the self*. London: Sage.
Maher, J. (2001). The promiscuous placenta: Crossing over. In A. Bashford & C. Hooker (eds) (pp. 201–216). *Contagion: Historical and cultural studies*. London: Routledge.
Maher, J., Fraser, S. & Wright, J. (2010). Framing the mother: Childhood obesity, maternal responsibility and care. *Journal of Gender Studies*, *19(3)*, 233–247.
Malik, H. (2007). *From placenta to lunchbox: Mothers, the media and fat kids*. Unpublished Honours Thesis. Bachelor of Physiotherapy, School of Health Sciences, University of South Australia.
McDowell, J. (2005). Plan health for future children. *South-East Advertiser Australia*, February 16.
McMillen, C., MacLaughlin, M., Muhlhausler, B., et al. (2008). Developmental origins of health and disease: The role of periconceptional and fetal nutrition. *Basic and Clinical Pharmacology and Toxicology*, *102*, 82–89.
McNaughton, D. (2011). From the womb to the tomb: Obesity and maternal responsibility. *Critical Public Health*, *21(2)*, 179–190.
Medew, J. (2009). Child neglect linked to feeding. *The Sydney Morning Herald*, 27 January, p. 3.
Moffat, T. (2010). The childhood obesity epidemic. *Medical Anthropology Quarterly*, *24(1)*, 1–21.
Monaghan, L., Holland, R. & Pritchard, G. (2010). Obesity epidemic entrepreneurs: Types, practices and interests. *Body & Society*, *16(2)*, 37–71.
Moore, V. & Davies, M. (2008). Early life influences on later health: The role of nutrition. *Asia Pacific Journal of Clinical Nutrition*, *10(2)*, 113–117.
Murray, S. (2005). (Un/Be)coming out? Rethinking fat politics. *Social Semiotics*, *15(2)*, 153–163.
Murray, S. (2008). Pathologising 'fatness': Medical authority and popular culture. *Sociology of Sport Journal*, *1*, 7–21.
Nerlich, B. (2009). The post-antibiotic apocalypse and the war on superbugs: Catastrophe discourse in microbiology, its rhetorical form and political function. *Public Understanding of Science*, *18(5)*, 574–590.
Oken, E. & Gillman, M. (2003). Fetal origins of obesity. *Obesity Research*, *11(4)*, 496–506.
Orbach, S. (2009). *Bodies*. London: Profile.
Parker, C. (2009). Where have all the 'good' mothers gone? Risk, responsibility and reproductive rights'. Paper presented to the 15th International Critical & Feminist Perspectives in Health and Social Justice Conference' Auckland University of Technology, Auckland, 17–19 April 2009.
Passamai-Inesedy, A. (2006). Confining risk: Choice and responsibility in childbirth in a risk society. *Health Sociology Review*, *15(4)*, 406–414.
Paul, A. (2010, September 22). How the first nine months shape the rest of your life. *Time Magazine*. Retrieved from http://www.time.com/time/health/article/0,8599,2020815,00.html.

Petchesky, R. (1987). Fetal images: The power of visual culture in the politics of reproduction. *Feminist Studies, 13(2)*, 263–292.
Petersen, A., Anderson, A., Allan, S. & Wilkinson, C. (2009). Opening the black box: Scientists views on the role of the news media in the nanotechnology debate. *Public Understanding of Science, 18(5)*, 512–530.
Ruddick, S. (2007). At the horizons of the subject: Neo-Liberalism, Neo-Conservatism and the rights of the child, part one. *Gender, Place and Culture, 14(5)*, 513–527.
Saguy, A. & Almeling, R. (2008). Fat in the fire? Science, the news media, and the obesity epidemic. *Sociological Forum, 23(1)*, 53–83.
ScienceDaily. (2007). Eating junk food while pregnant and breastfeeding may lead to obese offspring. *ScienceDaily*. Retrieved from http://www.sciencedaily.com /releases/2007/08/070814212154.htm [accessed June 16, 2011]
Shepherd, T. (2009). Overweight mums putting newborns at greater risk. *The Advertiser*, 16 March, p. 3.
Skeggs, B. (2005). The making of class through visualising moral subject formation. *Sociology, 39(5)*, 965–982.
Singh, I. (2004). Doing their jobs: Mothering with Ritalin in a culture of mother-blame. *Social Science & Medicine, 59*, 1193–1205.
Steele, S. (1999). A large legacy – overweight children may not have to look too far to find the reason – it could all be mum's fault. *Sunday Mail*, 7 November, p. 22.
Stewart, F. (2009). Mother's smoking gun. *The Advertiser*, 15 March, p. 11.
Susser, M. & Levin, B. (1999). Ordeals for the fetal programming hypothesis. *British Medical Journal, 318*, 885–886.
Taor, A. (2009). Breastfed children least likely to be abused by mothers. *The Australian*, 31 January, p. 5.
Unnithan-Kumar, M. (2011). Corporeality and reproduction: Understanding fatness through the diverse experiences of motherhood, consumption and social regulation. In M. Unnithan-Kumar & S. Tremane (eds), *Fatness and the maternal body: Women's experiences of corporeality and the shaping of social policy.* Oxford: Berghahn Books.
Ussher, J. (2006). *Managing the monstrous feminine: Regulating the reproductive body*. London and New York: Routledge.
Warin, M., Moore, V., Zivkovic, T. & Davies, M. (2011). Telescoping the origins of obesity to women's bodies: How gender inequalities are being squeezed out of Barker's Hypothesis. *Annals of Human Biology (Special Edition), 38(4)*, 453–60.
Wells, J. (2010). *The evolutionary biology of human body fatness: Thrift and control*. Cambridge Studies in Biological and Evolutionary Anthropology. Cambridge University Press.

Wright, J. & Harwood, V. (2009). *Biopolitics and the 'Obesity Epidemic': Governing bodies*. New York: Routledge.
Zivkovic, T., Warin, M., Davies, M. & Moore, V. (2010). In the name of the child: The gendered politics of childhood obesity. *Journal of Sociology*, *46*, 375–392.

Chapter 7
Eating Disorders in the Media: The Changing Nature of UK Newspaper Reports[1]

Emily Shepherd and Clive Seale

Introduction

Concerns about news reports of eating disorders have focused on the impact of reporting on public understanding of eating disorders. O'Hara and Clegg-Smith (2007) elaborate this view in their detailed study of eating disorder reporting in seven US newspapers during 2004–5. They call for journalists to improve coverage of the causality, medical complications and treatment modalities of eating disorders, to combat stereotypes that associate eating disorders exclusively with celebrities and younger white women, and to present eating disorders as medical diseases rather than outcomes of narcissistic dieting behaviour, curable by an effort of will.

In this chapter we report an investigation of UK newspaper reporting of eating disorders, first making a direct comparison with US media. Second, we track changes over a 17-year-period in a large sample of articles and third, we investigate differences between newspapers targeted at different social groups. Our findings suggest a re-evaluation of the role played by newspapers aimed at the 'popular' end of the newspaper market, and reveal a more complex picture of changing media messages than earlier studies.

Medical and Public Knowledge about Eating Disorders

Early medical evidence about the aetiology of eating disorders (Sassorili & Ruggiero, 2005) pointed to inner psychological factors (low self-esteem, high expectations of self and a stress response), social factors (cultural 'norms' of thinness as an ideal, media, advertising) and family factors (abuse, neglect and pressure from parents to achieve), together with other environmental influence, such as peer group norms (Eisenberg, Neumark-Sztainer, Story & Perry, 2005). But

1 Reprinted from Shepherd, E. & Seale, C. (2010). Eating disorders in the media: The changing nature of UK newspaper reports. *European Eating Disorders Review, 18(6)*, 486–495.

current medical thinking now stresses a view of eating disorders as multi-factorial complex mental diseases with genetic and biological as well as environmental roots (Bulik et al., 2006). Those with eating disorders are at higher risk of other psychological manifestations such as anxiety, obsessive compulsive disorder and depression (Staresinic, 2004). Medical complications associated with eating disorders include amenorrhoea, heart problems, osteoporosis and psychological dysfunction (Clinical Knowledge Summaries, 2009). Treatment includes medical therapy (antidepressants), psychological interventions and specialist inpatient care.

Evidence suggests public perceptions deviate from the medical view of eating disorders, both in the US (Global Market Insight, 2005) and in the UK (Crisp, 2005), with stigmatizing perceptions being prevalent, associated with a view that emphasizes eating disorders as the consequence of moral failings. These perceptions extend to some health care professionals, who are more likely to blame individuals for their eating disorder where socio-cultural causation, rather than biological/genetic causation, is foregrounded (Crisafulli, von Holle & Bulik, 2008). Stigmatization means that the experience of having an eating disorder is often associated with high levels of shame (Troop, Allan, Serpell & Treasure, 2008). Other evidence (O'Hara & Clegg-Smith, 2007) suggests lay people underestimate the severity and ease of recovery from eating disorders, as well as associating eating disorders almost exclusively with younger white women.

The Role of the Media

The role of the mass media in influencing the development of an eating disorder has been investigated far more extensively than the media portrayal of eating disorders themselves (Wykes & Gunter 2007). It has prompted much concern from policy makers and campaigning groups, and in the UK has led to government-sponsored attempts to regulate a prominent source of such media images of women: the fashion industry (Cussins, 2001). These regulatory moves are, of course, themselves reported widely in the media and further contribute to the public perception that eating disorders are caused by socio-cultural factors.

We are aware of only two studies of media portrayals of eating disorders. A study by Mondini, Favaro and Santonataso (1996) of Italian newspapers and magazines found that media stories tended to emphasize as causes socio-cultural factors (particularly ideal body images promoted by the fashion industry and the media themselves) and family dynamics (particularly parental influence). Medical complications of eating disorders were rarely reported and treatment was largely reported as involving psychotherapy, including psycho-analysis and family therapy.

O'Hara and Clegg-Smith (2007) studied 210 articles appearing in seven US newspapers between October 2004 and October 2005, largely focusing on stories containing personal profiles of individuals affected by anorexia or bulimia. These eating disorders were portrayed as arising from the struggle of individuals with the stress and low self-esteem caused by family dynamics and negative parental influence. Genetic or biological causation was mentioned in just two stories which did not link these to personal profiles. Profiles were largely of celebrities in the entertainment industry and younger white women. Clinical complications and medical treatments were rarely mentioned, recovery being shown as the outcome of willpower or chance event. The finding that 78 per cent of profiles showed successful recovery was regarded by these authors as unrealistic.

These authors describe eating disorder stories in newspapers as a 'source of titillation' and 'voyeuristic', failing to treat the subject as 'an issue that deserves serious consideration' and blurring the boundary between clinically diagnosed eating disorder and extreme dieting behaviour. They urge journalists to profile famous people with eating disorders who come from outside the entertainment industry, and people of different age, race and gender. More clinical information, so that newspaper accounts convey messages that are similar to medical perspectives, is also advocated.

Aims of this Study

We aimed to extend these existing studies of eating disorders in the media, first by examining coverage in a third country: the UK. Here, newspapers are more firmly divided into the national and local press than in the US and there is a clear segmentation of readerships amongst the nationals, with 'popular' or 'tabloid' newspapers catering for a less educated audience and having high circulation, and 'serious' or 'broadsheet' newspapers catering for the tastes of a more educated readership. As well as enabling direct comparisons with US newspapers, this segmentation of the newspaper market provided an opportunity to understand how media messages differ across different readerships.

The two existing studies reviewed above are limited to small samples and, in the case of O'Hara and Clegg-Smith (2007), to a single year of coverage. This results in an account of media content that is relatively static. In fact, media coverage changes over time as new stories develop and different sources are given prominence, so our study sought to track changes over a longer time period. Our aims in this study, then, are:

1. to describe messages about eating disorders conveyed in UK national newspaper reporting, and to compare this with the US.
2. to track changes over time, particularly regarding variations in the prominence of medical perspectives on eating disorders.
3. to differentiate coverage produced by different segments of the newspaper market, particularly with regard to the popular – serious distinction

By doing this, we hoped to make realistic recommendations about ways in which news reports may provide better public education about the nature of eating disorders and less stigmatizing coverage.

Methods

The study contained three linked investigations, each of which will be described in turn.

Investigation 1: Comparison with US Newspapers

The *Nexis* database was used to retrieve 205 newspaper articles appearing in seven UK newspapers between 13 October 2004 and 13 October 2005 containing the terms '*anore!*' OR '*bulim!*' OR '*eating disorder*' (where ! is a 'wildcard' character and searches for all variants of the word: e.g., *anorexia/xic/ctic*). These replicate procedures used by O'Hara and Clegg-Smith (2007). The newspapers chosen were the *Times, Telegraph, Independent* and *Guardian* (all 'serious'), the *Sun* and *Mirror* (popular) and the *Daily Mail*, which targets a largely female readership and stands between serious and popular in its emphases.

Seventy-three full personal profiles and 68 brief mentions of someone with an eating disorder were identified in these articles. A coding scheme was applied to these profiles and a separate blind intercoder reliability exercise covering 28 full personal profiles resulted in a kappa statistic of 0.779.

Investigation 2: Time Trends

Articles in *Nexis* appearing between 1992 and 2008 (inclusive) were retrieved, using the same search terms as in Investigation 1. The *Sun, Mirror* and *Telegraph* were not uploaded by 1992 so were excluded from this sample. The 2,355 articles retrieved in this way were analysed using *Wordsmith Tools* for comparative keyword analysis (Seale & Charteris-Black, 2010; Seale, Charteris-Black & Ziebland, 2006) to track changes in eating disorder coverage over four time periods: *1992–1996*; *1997–2000*; *2001–2004*; *2005–2008.*

Investigation 3: Popular and Serious Newspapers

Articles in *Nexis* appearing between 2001 and 2008 (inclusive) were retrieved, using the same search terms and same newspapers as in Investigation 1, excluding the *Daily Mail*. The sample was divided into:

a. Serious (*Times*, *Telegraph*, *Guardian*, *Independent*, in which 524 articles appeared);
b. Popular (*Sun*, *Mirror*; 519 articles).

Wordsmith Tools was used to track the usage of key terms relating to aetiology, clinical complications, treatment, and other terms which were identified as important themes in coverage during investigations 1 and 2 (see Table 7.3).

Table 7.1 Comparison between US and UK national newspapers: Personal profiles of people with eating disorders

	US [1]	UK full profiles	UK brief profiles	All UK profiles	P value[a]
Female	95/100 (95%)	66/72 (92%)	60/69 (87%)	126/141 89%)	$p = 0.118$
Age at onset					
Pre-teen, teen or college student	57/100 (57%)	46/66 (70%)	27/63 (43%)	73/129 (57%)	
Young adult (20s)	25/100 (25%)	14/66 (21%)	24/63 (38%)	38/129 (29%)	$p = 0.1225$
Over 30	18/100 (18%)	3/66 (5%)	8/63 (13%)	11/129 (9%)	
White	48/51 (94%)	41/42 (98%)	53/58 (91%)	94/100 (94%)	$p = 0.642$
Celebrity	–	31/72 (43%)	50/69 (75%)	81/141 (58%)	–
Aetiology					
Mentioned at all[b]	33/100 (33%)	34/72 (47%)	20/69 (29%)	54/141 (38%)	$p = 0.399$[b]
Family dynamics	16/100 (16%)	17/72 (24%)	12/69 (17%)	29/141 (21%)	$p = 0.37$
Psychological	–	27/72 (38%)	16/69 (23%)	43/141 (30%)	–
Genetic/biological	0/100 (0%)	2/72 (3%)	6/69 (9%)	8/141 (6%)	$p = 0.013$[c]
Other	–	36/72 (50%)	8/69 (12%)	44/141 (31%)	–
Clinical complications	11/100 (11%)	47/72 (65%)	21/69 (30%)	68/141 (48%)	$p < 0.0001$
Physical	–	39/72 (54%)	15/69 (22%)	54/141 (38%)	–
Psychological	–	27/72 (38%)	6/69 (9%)	33/141 (23%)	–
Treatment mentioned at all	21/100 (21%)	40/72 (56%)	22/69 (32%)	62/141 (44%)	$p = 0.0002$
Medical	–	11/72 (15%)	11/69 (16%)	22/141 (16%)	–
Psychological	–	22/72 (31%)	11/69 (16%)	3/141 (23%)	–
Medical or psychological	8/100 (8%)	24/72 (33%)	12/69 (18%)	36/141 (26%)	$p = 0.0005$
Hospitalization	0/100 (0%)	24/72 (33%)	10/69 (14%)	34/141 (24%)	$p < 0.0001$[c]
Had recovered	78/100 (78%)	20/72[d] (28%)	26/69[d] (38%)	46/141[d] (33%)	$p < 0.0001$
N	100	72	69	141	

Note: a – For comparison of US and all UK profiles, based on χ^2 test; b – Comparison of only family dynamics and genetic/biological aetiology; c – Based on Fisher's exact test; d – UK figures exclude Princess Diana because her recovery status at the time of her death is unclear.

Results

Investigation 1: Comparison with US Newspapers

Table 7.1 shows how UK and US coverage compares, for personal profiles. For demographic variables (gender, age, race) coverage is similar. The focus on celebrities noted in the US study (but not coded and counted) is also considerable in the UK. Coverage of aetiology is similar with the exception of genetic/biological causation, which entered only two non-profile articles in the US study, but entered four non-profile articles in the UK and a further eight profiles. The clinical complications of eating disorders are four times as likely to be discussed in the UK press and treatments are twice as likely to be reported, including hospitalization. Recovery from eating disorders is much less likely to be depicted in the UK press sample. Box 7.1 shows extracts illustrating some of these themes. It appears UK reporting of eating disorders contains more medical information and a less optimistic picture of the prospects for recovery than US newspaper coverage.

Box 7.1 Examples of UK newspaper discussion of eating disorders in 2004–2005

a) Celebrity stories: 'Prolonged starvation can lead to infertility and osteoporosis. In some cases, people with the disease die from the effects. Singers Karen Carpenter – the first "celebrity" anorexic – and Lena Zavaroni both fought long battles with anorexia and died young; Karen aged 32 and Lena aged 35'. *Daily Mail*, September 2005

b) Genetic and biological factors: 'People with anorexia and bulimia share core traits that are genetically based, claim studies in the online edition of *The American Journal of Medical Genetics Part B*'. *Times*, September 2005

c) Complications and treatment: 'With that kind of weight loss they have bone marrow and hormone suppression. Due to their starvation, their metabolism shuts down (and) they can just drop dead from a heart attack'. *Mirror*, May 2005

'Experts hope the new results will help to accelerate the search for potential treatments. Traditionally they have centred on psychotherapy, nutrition and, in some cases, medication such as antidepressants'. *Daily Mail*, September 2005

d) Recovery: 'Around four in ten patients fully recover, and many more live with the disease in a less acute form. The more we know about this disease, the more likely it is that we will one day find a cure'. *Daily Mail*, September 2005

Table 7.2 Keyword comparison over time of UK newspapers

1992–96	1997–2000	2001–2004	2005–2008
1. Fashion			
NONE	model/s; fashion	NONE	model/s; fashion week/industry/ council; BFC (British Fashion Council); (size) zero; Madrid; Milan; Spanish; catwalk; designers; Donatella (Versace); Reston/Ramos (models)
2. Medical terminology			
Slimming (disease/pact); bulimia	eating (disorders); operation	eating disorder; ED; health/y; CR (calorie restrictor); diabetes; levels – hormone/blood sugar; bone; study	eating disorder; BMI (body mass)index; health/y; CBT; experts; orthorexia; pregnancy; diabetes; risk
3. Internet			
	www	www; org; com; websites; pro(ana); internet	www; org; com; websites; pro ana; online; internet; (miss) bimbo
*4. Official concern and regulation**			
Conference; (Mrs)Penney	Summit; BMA; (Tessa) Jowell; (Peggy) Claude-Pierre	NONE	ban/ned; (model health) inquiry; chief (executive); (Lady) Kingsmill; Jowell; Eating Disorder Association
5. Celebrity sufferers			
Diana; Karen Carpenter; Audrey Hepburn; Britt Ekland; Elton John; Isabella (Hervey)	Lena Zavaroni; Spice (Girls); Posh; (Victoria) Beckham; Geri (Halliwell); Tracy (Shaw); Monica (Seles); Calista Flockhart; Ally (McBeal); Sophie (Dahl); Sophie (Anderton)	Geri Halliwell; Spice (Girls); Sandra (Dee); Celine (Dion); Maxine Carr; (Victoria) Beckham; Tracy (Shaw); Tara (Palmer-Tomkinson); (Daniela) Hantuchova; Rory (Bremner); Lara (Flynne-Boyle)	(John) Prescott; (Victoria) Beckham; Geri (Halliwell); Posh Spice; Spice Girls; Keira Knightley; Nicole Richie; Gail (Porter); (Jo) Brand; Allegra (Versace); Maxine (Carr); Edie Sedgwick; Debs (Deborah Barham); Billie (Piper); Sandra (Dee); Cheeky (Girls); (Teri) Hatcher

Table 7.2 continued

6. *Royal words*			
1992–1996	**1997–2000**	**2001–2004**	**2005–2008**
Princess Diana; Prince Charles; William; MB (Martin Bashir); HRH; Queen; monarchy; royal; palace; Wales; Windsor; Countess; Earl Spencer; Camilla Bowles; Johnnie Raine; (Andrew) Morton; (Susie) Orbach;	Chantal Collopy; Gauntlett; (Lawyer); Cape (Town)**	(Paul) Burrell	NONE

Note: Times, *Independent*, *Guardian* and *Daily Mail*; * Mrs Penney was president of the Girls' School Association; Tessa Jowell was the Minister for Women; Peggy Claude-Pierre founded the Montreux Clinic in Canada; Lady Kingsmill was the chairman of the Model Health Inquiry; ** Chantal Collopy was Earl Spencer's mistress; Gauntlett is the surname of Lady Spencer's lawyer; Cape Town is where Diana's brother lived.

Investigation 2: Time Trends

Table 7.2 displays the results of a keyword comparison of four time periods. For the first five categories (fashion, medical terminology, internet, official concern and regulation, celebrity sufferers) this was produced by making four separate comparisons:

1. The words in the '05–08' column are appear more frequently in articles published between 1 January 2005 and 31 December 2008, when compared with articles published between the same months in 1992–1996 (the 'reference category' for this comparison).
2. The words in the '01–04' column are those appearing most frequently at this point in time again compared with the 92–96 reference category. This is also true for the words in the '97–00' column.
3. The words in the '92–96' column are those appearing most frequently at that time across all the above comparisons.

The sixth and final row ('Royal words') follows the same logic but uses "05–08" as the reference category. Words given in parentheses are either the common collocations of the terms in the table which explain their predominant meaning, or expand shortened forms. The statistical cut-off point for including a word as a 'keyword' was $p < 0.000001$, based on a log-likelihood test. Keywords not belonging to the categories in the table are not shown.

In the earliest years of this coverage, Royal words are particularly prominent. This reflects the fact that reporting on eating disorders received a massive boost when Diana, princess of Wales, revealed her difficulties with eating and bulimia to the journalists Andrew Morton and Martin Bashir, and the subsequent coverage which included Susie Orbach, Diana's therapist and author of the book *Fat is a Feminist Issue* (1978). Table 7.2 shows that the connection with Diana declines over time, but that press interest in an ever-changing cast of celebrities with eating disorders remains a constant, most of whom are figures in the entertainment industry, with the notable exceptions of John Prescott, a government minister, and Maxine Carr, convicted for a crime, in the latest period. Tracking the growth of the internet during this period, references to websites increase, with stories about the dangers of pro-anorexia sites and others felt to encourage extreme dieting becoming more common in the later period.

Box 7.2 shows extracts from news coverage containing these themes, as well as extracts which illustrate the emergence of concern about images of super thin models in the fashion industry. Table 7.2 shows this to be more common in later years of coverage, and the vocabulary of official concern and regulation of this industry is particularly prominent in the latest time period.

Box 7.2 Three themes that have changed over time in UK newspaper reporting of eating disorders

a) Royal reporting: 'The Princess of Wales is to visit a conference on life-threatening eating disorders. It will be the first time that Diana, who is widely believed to have suffered from the bingeing disorder bulimia nervosa, has publicly shown her concern about the problem'. *Daily Mail*, January 1993

b) The internet: 'The mental health charity Sane is currently conducting research into pro-anorexia websites and preliminary findings show that almost three-quarters of those visiting them had experienced suicidal thoughts or feelings, while almost half said they self-harmed'. *Guardian*, July 2006

c) The fashion industry, official concern and regulation: 'Of course, we have all been here before. In June 2000, I co-chaired a Body Summit with Tessa Jowell, then minister for women, at which we asked representatives from the fashion industry if they would not at least be sensible and introduce a BMI cut-off point'. *Daily Mail*, February 2007

Table 7.2 also shows a marked increase over time in medical terminology, and Box 7.3 shows examples of this coverage. The term 'slimming disease' in earlier coverage (coupled with the 'bulimia' said to have been experienced by Princess Diana) is superseded in later coverage with the medical term 'eating disorder', in part because of the emergence of the Eating Disorders Association, increasingly consulted by journalists. Terms such as BMI (body mass index) and CBT (cognitive behaviour therapy) have in later years become part of press vocabulary associated with eating disorders. The consequences of eating disorders, particularly the risk of diabetes when overweight, is more commonly discussed in the later years.

Investigation 3: Popular and Serious Papers

Table 7.3 compares frequencies of words and clusters of words between popular and serious newspapers. As one might expect, reports of 'research' are significantly more common in the serious papers, as are stories about genetic causation of eating disorders, which tend to be reported as scientific research stories. However, interpersonal and socio-cultural aetiological factors show no difference between popular and serious papers and the same is true of words describing most treatments.

Box 7.3 Medical terminology in UK newspaper reports of eating disorders

a) CBT: 'One approach she has tried over the past few years, and continues to be treated with regularly, is cognitive behavioural therapy (CBT), a "talking" therapy which was largely ignored until 10 years ago but which, as well as being used as treatment for bulimics, is suddenly being touted as the best "evidence-based" (i.e. rigorously scientifically tested) cure for just about everything, from depression and phobias to schizophrenia, ME, obsessive compulsive disorder and obesity'. *Guardian*, June 2006

b) BMI: '12.5 (the) BMI of Ana Carolina Reston, the Brazilian model who died of anorexia in 2006. She was two and a half stone below the recommended minimum weight for her height'. *The Times*, April 2008

c) Orthorexia: 'regimens can vary wildly from person to person, with many orthorexics being, for instance, raw foodists, vegans, fruitarians or, in one notable case … committed to eating only yellow foods'. *Mail*, April 2007

Table 7.3 Frequency* of common words, by type of newspaper: 2001–2008

Words	Popular press	Serious press	Significance (based on log-likelihood)
Aetiology: ('abuse'; 'parental'; 'pressure'; expectations'; 'self-esteem'; [media/celebrity] 'influen!')	2.3	1.7	n.s.
'gene!'	0.2	0.9	$p < 0.0001$
'research'	2.9	7.5	$p < 0.0001$
Clinical complications: ('periods'; 'menstru!' 'thyroid/xine'; 'hair'; 'anaemia/c'; 'heart'; 'osteoporosis/tic'; 'bone/s'; 'brittle'; 'kidney/s')	21.2	11.8	$p < 0.0001$
Treatment: ('Cognitive behavioural therapy' or 'CBT'; 'psych!'; 'rehab'; 'clinic')	2.9	3.5	n.s.
'hospital' (ized/s)	10.9	5.8	$p < 0.0001$
Fashion industry and regulation: ('fashion'; (fashion/modelling) 'industry'; 'catwalk!'; 'model!' 'ban/ned')	13.6	42.6	$p < 0.0001$
Internet words: ('Pro-ana/mia'; 'web/site')	1.6	3.1	$p < 0.0001$
Celebrity: 'Diana'	2.2	1.0	$p < 0.0001$
Total words	357,537	496,694	

Note: * per 10,000 words.

The greater interest shown in clinical complications and hospitals by popular papers goes against expectations. This therefore prompted further investigation. The popular newspaper usage of 'hospital' was found to be commonly associated

Box 7.4 Medical information in popular and serious newspapers

Aetiology: POPULAR: 'Healthier-looking girls will be a better image for the many young women who develop eating disorders, influenced by images of skeletal models'. *Sun*, July 2007

POPULAR: 'Dear Deidre, I'm a 21-year-old girl ... I force food into my mouth even when I feel I can eat no more. I live with my parents and they stop me eating outside meal times but I find excuses to go out and buy food. DEIDRE SAYS: ... Though you are an adult, your parents seem to be running your life – or trying to. The emotional battle is really for your independence'. *Sun*, November 2003

Genetics: SERIOUS: 'Both sets of results point to a strong genetic component to anorexia and bulimia and an underlying biological reason why some girls are more prone to developing eating disorders than others'. *Independent*, March 2001

Research: SERIOUS: 'More than 500 teenagers took part in the study, carried out by the Centre of Appearance Research at the University of the West of England. The study assessed pressure from parents, siblings, friends and the media to be thin'. *Independent*, May 2006

Clinical complications: POPULAR: 'Looking in the mirror, I saw a skeletal mess. I had so little body fat it was uncomfortable to sit or even lie down. My periods had stopped and I was so cold, I needed to layer on jumpers, socks and even a hot-water bottle'. *Mirror*, November 2007

POPULAR: 'I was told I had ruined my chances of having children. And I was now too weak to hold down my job. There was nothing going for me ... I was sent for psychiatric treatment. I just couldn't seem to conquer this at all. The acid from persistent vomiting rotted my teeth. I stopped socialising. My entire life revolved around food and my revulsion to it'. *Sun*, February 2005

Treatment: SERIOUS: 'Ulrike Schmidt, consultant psychiatrist at the Maudsley Hospital and Professor of Eating Disorders at the Institute of Psychiatry at King's College London, said: "In five years we hope to have new treatments for anorexia that make a lasting and positive difference to sufferers and their families"'. *Times*, April 2007

with events happening to individuals whose personal stories were being told, some of whom were 'rushed into hospital' or went 'in and out of hospital'. By contrast, in the serious papers, 37 per cent of the use of 'hospital' referred to the names of specific hospitals such as 'St Georges Hospital', 'The Priory Hospital', 'Great Ormond St Hospital' and 'The Maudsley Hospital', compared to 7 per cent of mentions in the popular papers. In addition, further analysis of the sample used in Investigation 1 showed that popular papers were more likely to profile individuals than serious papers (61 per cent of popular news articles in this sample involved profiles, as opposed to 47 per cent of serious news articles). This is confirmed by the finding for 'Diana' in Table 7.3. The description of the harrowing clinical complications experienced by profiled individuals with eating disorders was used to increase their emotional impact (see also Box 7.4).

Discussion

In both the US and the UK there is a consistent association of eating disorders with younger white women and celebrities, largely caused by interpersonal and socio-cultural factors. But in the UK, genetic and biological causation is somewhat more frequently reported, and it is more common to portray eating disorders as serious illness with clinical complications requiring medical treatment, including hospitalization. UK coverage is more pessimistic than US coverage about the prospects of recovery from eating disorders, a finding consistent with the reporting of cancer experience in North American newspapers, where stories of bravery, recovery and survivorship predominate (Seale, 2002).

Our comparison of the popular and serious press (Investigation 3) suggests an explanation for this. The UK newspaper scene is markedly driven by a popular or 'tabloid' agenda (McLachlan & Golding, 2000), where personal profiles are an important vehicle for news reporters. To increase emotional impact, harrowing stories with often lurid accounts of clinical complications and hospital admissions are published. Thus the popular press is more likely to carry such information, contrasting with the expectation that the serious press might present more medical details of eating disorders.

Serious UK newspapers have traditionally been the platform for political news, science stories and issues affecting public health (see, for example, Seale, Boden, Lowe, et al., 2007), with the popular press predominantly reporting stories about sex and scandal. Some of our findings support this view, with serious newspapers focusing more on stories about research and genetic causation of eating disorders, about the dangers of the internet, the regulation of the fashion industry, and less celebrity gossip or Royal stories. But our study cautions against the view that a populist agenda undermines the capacity of newspapers to present medical information, as the popular press in the UK is the vehicle for considerable emphasis on the serious nature of eating disorders, and on their status as diseases deserving medical attention.

Our second investigation, of trends over time, shows that news about eating disorders is not static. Beginning with an overwhelming emphasis on news about Princess Diana's bulimia in the earliest period we studied, the story developed over time to incorporate a range of other concerns. In part, this was a response to the emergence of new and influential voices in the public concern about eating disorders, such as the Eating Disorders Association which, like other awareness-raising organizations, sought media publicity for its views. High profile political involvement in concern about the socio-cultural causation of eating disorders led to the emergence of stories about attempts to regulate the fashion industry. Journalists therefore had to seek out new sources, so that what was originally a royal story became increasingly a public health and, to some extent, a science story. Through these processes medical terminology has increasingly entered media discourse, arguably producing coverage that is more in line with the view of eating disorders as diseases with complex causative factors, requiring medical and psychological treatment.

In one respect, though, UK newspapers lag behind medical opinion. Genetic and biological causation is largely treated as a stand-alone science story and is not well integrated into personal profiles. Of 12 articles which referred to genetic or biological causation in the sample studied in our first investigation, only two appeared in full personal profiles. If it is accepted that public education is best achieved by providing medical information in a popular format, it might be argued that journalists should find a way to include such information in personal profiles. This has been achieved, for example, in the media coverage of breast cancer genetics (Henderson & Kitzinger, 1999).

In addition, it should be noted that our study includes only newspapers. Magazines, broadcast media and the internet are sources on which people draw for information about health issues. Studies of information about eating disorders provided by these sources would extend and deepen understanding. Understanding how members of media audiences incorporate – and sometimes resist – messages from the media in their everyday lives also requires a different kind of study. The intentions of media producers, and the apparent messages contained in media content, do not always translate smoothly into public understanding (Hall, 1980).

Conclusion

Using several methods of text analysis and different comparison groups we have been able to go beyond a static account of a small, time-limited sample of news articles. We have shown how national newspaper cultures sometimes differ, how the eating disorder story has changed over time, and how different segments of the newspaper industry provide variations in reporting styles and content. The picture we reveal is far from being a simple story of media sensationalism. We argue for a more realistic appreciation of the constraints on journalists and a better understanding of the popular entertainment format with which so many of them work.

Numerous studies of mass media reporting of science and medical stories focus on their tendency to sensationalize or to produce health-damaging effects (Seale, 2003). We take the view that fixing this by making media stories more like reports in medical journals may appear an obvious solution, but is unappealing to journalists whose agenda prioritizes entertainment and sales above public education. The media sensationalize and simplify because this works on the emotions of readers more effectively than the presentation of complex scientific information. Personal profile stories involving celebrities have much more currency – particularly at the 'popular' end of the newspaper market – than reports of scientific knowledge. For these reasons, 'edutainment', social marketing and media advocacy have arisen as health promotion strategies that recognize and adapt to these media realities (Naidoo & Wills, 2009). The 'soft' news item involving celebrity gossip in a popular media outlet may be a better vehicle for public education than a 'hard' news item on scientific discovery in a 'serious' newspaper.

References

Bulik, C.M., Sullivan, P.F., Tozzi, F., et al. (2006). Prevalence, heritability, and prospective risk factors for anorexia nervosa. *Archives of General Psychiatry*, *63*, 305–312.

Clinical Knowledge Summaries, National Library for Health. (2009). *Eating disorders.* Retrieved from www.cks.library.nhs.uk/eating_disorders/background _information [accessed September 18, 2009].

Crisafulli, M.A., von Holle, A. & Bulik, C.M. (2008). Attitudes towards anorexia nervosa: The impact of framing on blame and stigma. *International Journal of Eating Disorders*, *41*, 333–339.

Crisp, A. (2005). Stigmatization of and discrimination against people with eating disorders including a report of two nationwide surveys. *European Eating Disorders Review*, *53*, 147–152.

Cussins, A.M. (2001). The role of body image in women's mental health. *Feminist Review*, 68, 105–114.

Eisenberg, M.E., Neumark-Sztainer, D., Story, M. & Perry, C. (2005). The role of social norms and friends' influences on unhealthy weight-control behaviors among adolescent girls. *Social Science & Medicine*, *60*, 1165–1173.

Global Market Insight (2005). American public opinion on eating disorders: Poll conducted on behalf of the National Eating Disorders Association. Seattle: GMI Inc. Retrieved from www.nationaleatingdisorders.org/nedaDir%5Cfiles %5Cdocuments%5CGMIcollege.pdf [accessed September 18, 2009].

Hall, S. (1980). Encoding/decoding. In S. Hall, *Culture, media, language* (pp. 128–138). London: Hutchinson.

Henderson, L. & Kitzinger, J. (1999). The human drama of genetics: 'Hard' and 'soft' media representations of inherited breast cancer. *Sociology of Health & Illness*, 21, 560–578.

McLachlan, S. & Golding, P. (2000). Tabloidisation in the British press: A quantitative investigation into changes in British newspapers, 1952–1997. In C. Sparks & J. Tulloch (eds), *Tabloid tales: Global debates over media standards* (pp. 76–90). London: Rowman and Littlefield.

Mondini, S., Favaro, A. & Santonataso, P. (1996). Eating disorders and the ideal of feminine beauty in Italian newspapers and magazines. *European Eating Disorders Review*, *4*, 112–120.

Naidoo, J. & Wills, J. (2009). *Foundations for health promotion* (3rd edition). Oxford: Baillière Tindall.
O'Hara, S.K. & Clegg Smith, K. (2007). Presentation of eating disorders in the news media: What are the implications for patient diagnosis and treatment? *Patient Education and Counselling, 68*, 43–51.
Orbach, S. (1978). *Fat is a feminist issue*. London: Paddington Books.
Sassorili, S. & Ruggiero, G.M. (2005). The role of stress in the association between low self-esteem, perfectionism, and worry, and eating disorders. *International Journal of Eating Disorders, 37*, 135–141.
Seale, C., Boden, S., Lowe, P., et al. (2007). Media constructions of sleep and sleep disorders: A study of UK national newspapers. *Social Science & Medicine, 65*, 418–430.
Seale, C., Charteris-Black, J. & Ziebland, S. (2006). Gender, cancer experience and internet use: A comparative keyword analysis of interviews and online cancer support groups. *Social Science & Medicine, 62*, 2577–2590.
Seale, C. & Charteris-Black, J. (2010). Keyword analysis: A new tool for qualitative research. In I.L. Bourgeault, R. DeVries, R. Dingwall (eds), *Handbook of qualitative health research.* Thousand Oaks, CA: Sage.
Seale, C. (2002). Cancer heroics: A study of news reports with particular reference to gender. *Sociology, 36*, 107–126.
Seale, C. (2003). *Media and health.* London: Sage.
Staresinic, C. (2004). Refusing sustenance. *PittMed*, May, 13–16.
Troop, N.A., Allan, S., Serpell, L. & Treasure, J.L. (2008). Shame in women with a history of eating disorders. *European Eating Disorders Review, 16*, 480–488.
Wykes, M. & Gunter, B. (2007). *The media and body image*. London: Sage.

Chapter 8
Making the 'Obesity Epidemic': The Role of Science and the News Media[1]

Abigail C. Saguy and Rene Almeling

Obesity is the 'terror within', according to Surgeon General Richard Carmona who says that 'unless we do something about it, the magnitude of the dilemma will dwarf 9/11 or any other terrorist attempt' (Associated Press, 2006). This statement reflects two decades of increasingly intense concern that America is eating itself to death. The alarm over body weight is based on current definitions in which anyone with a Body Mass Index (BMI, weight in kilos divided by height in meters squared) over 25 is deemed "overweight" and anyone with a BMI over 30 is labelled 'obese'. By these definitions, an average height woman (5'4") is 'overweight' at 146 pounds and 'obese' at 175 pounds, while a man of average height (5'9") is 'overweight' at 170 pounds and 'obese' at 203 pounds. Over one half of the US population in the 1960s and almost 2/3 of the US population today weigh 'too much' by these standards (Flegal et al., 2005; Flegal et al., 2002; Kuczmarski, 1994).

Some researchers have argued concern over an obesity epidemic is overblown and misguided (Ernsberger & Haskew, 1987; Gaesser, 1996; Campos, 2004; Campos et al., 2006; Oliver, 2005). A 2005 study by scientists at the Centers for Disease Control and Prevention (CDC) suggested that it is only after BMI reaches 35 that there is a meaningful increase in mortality, and that people in the 'overweight' category (BMI between 25 and 30) actually have the lowest rate of mortality (Flegal et al., 2005). This chapter does not seek to intervene in these debates. Rather, in the tradition of the sociology of social problems (Spector and Kitsuse, 1977), we aim to shed light on how 'overweight' and 'obesity' are being defined by claims-makers as social problems. Examining the claims-making activities of scientific research and the news media and interactions between them, this chapter builds on other work that has examined how weight has been framed by medical professionals, researchers, fat acceptance activists, the CDC, and a food industry lobby called the Center for Consumer Freedom (CCF) (Sobal, 1995; Saguy & Riley, 2005; Kwan, 2009).

As patients become more likely to seek medical information directly (Schlesinger, 2002), they are more likely to get their information from news

1 This is a shortened version of Saguy, A.C. & Almeling, R. (2008). Fat in the fire? Science, the news media, and the 'Obesity Epidemic'. *Sociological Forum, 23(1)*, 53–83.

sources than from scientific studies (Nelkin, 1987; Carlsson, 2000). It is thus increasingly important to understand how the mass media 'filter and translate scientific information' (Epstein, 1996: 22). In addition to information, the news media convey social norms and hierarchies as well, making them an important research site for cultural sociologists. Body weight and eating have traditionally been subject to moral connotations as indicators of sloth and gluttony (see Lyman, 1989). An additional layer of morality has been added to body weight and eating as controlled appetite and trim bodies have come to represent healthy living, in a society where the pursuit of health is a moral end in itself (Crawford, 1980).

This chapter speaks to the long-standing interest among feminist scholars in the pressures on women to conform to narrowly defined and unrealistic body expectations (Bordo, 1993; Wolf, 1991). Feminists have criticized the fashion industry for promoting images of ultra-thin female bodies, which encourage women to lose weight (Bordo, 1993; Chernin, 1995; Media Education Foundation, 1999; Thompson, 1994; Wolf, 1991) and purchase products or undergo regiments that promise weight loss, even when they prove ineffective (Bish et al., 2005; Santry et al., 2005; Fraser, 1998). Fat acceptance activists have written about fat women's experience of fat-hatred in contemporary societies (Wann, 1999; Cooper, 1998; Schoenfielder & Wieser, 1983, see also Millman, 1980). Our study builds on this work by being the first to examine the respective role of medical expertise and medical reporting in shaping normative understandings of body weight.

Intersecting with these gendered discourses about body weight are racial and class inequalities. Middle-class white girls have been more vulnerable to feeling that they could never be 'thin enough' (Hesse-Biber, 1996) and to the eating disorders and negative body image that ensue from that sentiment. In contrast, African-American girls seemed relatively better off, with positive self-image – even at higher weights – a product of affirming messages prevalent in African-American communities about individual style and respect for one's body (Nichter, 2000). However, increasing public health attention to 'epidemic rates of obesity' among African-Americans, as well as Mexican-Americans, and the poor means that positive body-image at higher weights among women and girls in these groups is being increasingly portrayed as socially irresponsible and unhealthy.

Drawing on a sample of scientific studies, press releases on those studies, and news reports on those same studies, we compare how the medical implications of body weight are framed differently across these three kinds of texts. We ask what role the news media, compared to scientific publications, play in framing obesity as a public health crisis. Do journalists sensationalize work on which they are reporting? Do they colour morally-neutral scientific accounts with moral overtones or, alternatively, are they merely reflecting the moral condemnations of fatness in the original studies? What themes, metaphors, or language, if any, are journalists and editors introducing that are absent from the original studies on which they are reporting? What role do press releases play in translating science into news? The analysis contributes to understanding how overweight and obesity are being constructed as medical and public health problems, and more generally, how science informs news reporting on health risks and health crises.

Framing Body Weight

By framing, we mean the selection and emphasis of 'some aspects of a perceived reality ... in such a way as to promote a particular problem definition' (Entman, 1993: 52). The terms 'overweight' and 'obesity' are themselves powerful and contested frames for understanding higher body weight as either a risk factor for disease or a disease in itself. Body weight is thus 'medicalized' (Conrad & Schneider, 1992), rather than being treated as a political or civil rights issue, as other claims-makers argue it should be (Wann, 1999; LeBesco, 2004; Cooper, 1998; see Sobal, 1995; Saguy & Riley, 2005). Fat acceptance activists reject the terms 'overweight' and 'obesity' because they reject the medical framing of higher body weights. Instead they reclaim the term 'fat' to speak of larger bodies as part of a natural and desirable form of diversity (Saguy & Riley, 2005).

Research on framing shows that different media frames imply not only different ways of understanding social problems but also different courses of action (Gamson, 1992; Snow & Benford, 1988; Tarrow, 1992). If fatness is framed as a natural and desirable form of biological diversity, this suggests that we should promote greater social tolerance. If, on the other hand, fatness is framed as the product of unhealthy choices, fat people (and ethnic groups with higher population weights) are likely to be cast as morally deviant or even 'villain' (Gusfield, 1981). Influential epidemiological studies have framed obesity as a 'preventable' cause of illness, much like smoking (Mokdad et al., 2004), and leading obesity researchers also tend to rely on a 'risky behavior' framing of fatness (Saguy & Riley, 2005). When speaking of childhood obesity, 'parents who do nothing to prevent obesity in their children' may be considered 'guilty of abuse, if not legally then morally' (Lovric, 2005). Various claims-makers have framed 'obesity' as a dire public health threat or 'epidemic' in order to promote investment of public funds into research and treatment or to relax safeguards against the risks of weight-loss treatments, drugs, or surgery (Saguy & Riley, 2005; Oliver, 2005).

Some argue that medicalizing body weight lessens the moral blame associated with fatness (Sobal, 1995; see also Conrad & Scheider, 1992). However, while framing obesity as a disease outside of individual control might remove blame, it reinforces the stigma (Goffman, 1963) associated with fatness in that it relies on an understanding of fatness as diseased (Saguy & Riley, 2005). An alternative framing of this issue blames the food industry or car culture for contributing to an 'obesogenic' environment (see Linn, 2004; Tartamella, Herscher & Woolston, 2005; Dalton, 2004; Nestle, 2002; Brownell & Horgen, 2003). Some have argued that this environmental frame lessens individual blame (Lawrence, 2003). We consider this an empirical question, but we are skeptical because, as Sylvia Noble Tesh (1988: 56) has commented: '[When an environmental theory of disease causality] refers mostly to smoking, eating and other forms of behaviour, then the responsibility for disease [remains] largely personal'.

Science and News Reporting: Dramatizing and Moralizing

Institutionalized mechanisms lead both scientists and journalists to dramatize and moralize. Scientists have an incentive to dramatize in a context where 'the language of crisis and imminent doom seem in a mass society to be the only way to get anyone's attention' (Edgley & Brissett, 1990: 268). Epidemiology takes the individual as the unit of analysis, just as 'healthism situates the problem of health and disease at the level of the individual with solutions formulated at that level as well' (Edgley & Brissett, 1990: 159). Belief in health as 'both an individual responsibility and a moral obligation', further provides 'a justification for meddling into the lives of those persons who seem either ignorant of that "fact" or unable or unwilling to act on it' (Edgley & Brissett, 1990: 259).

Commercial pressures also lead the news media dramatization (Bennett, 1983). Science journalists have been shown to favour imagery over content, cover research as a series of dramatic events, and report on provocative theory as if it were fact (Nelkin, 1987: 30; Gieryn & Figert, 1990). The common use by journalists of metaphors like 'epidemic' or 'war' to attract attention to social problems (see Darnton, 1975; see Calasanti & Slevin, 2001: 55; Clark & Everest, 2006) further contributes to alarmist reporting. Moreover, news reporting tends to be 'people-centred', where 'clearly identified individuals personify or stand in for larger, more difficult to grasp social forces', and 'news tends to simplify complex social processes in ways that emphasize melodrama, that turn a complex set of phenomenon into a morality tale' (Schudson, 2003: 48). In that most contemporary US journalists lack the time to do investigative and critical reporting, news sources exert a great deal of influence (Schudson, 2003; Tuchman, 1978; Gans, 1979; Ericson et al., 1989). Science reporting is expected to be especially uncritical and reliant on scientists due to reverence for science, complexity of materials, and lack of scientific training (Nelkin, 1987).

This literature informs our four central questions: 1) Do the news media dramatize more than the scientific studies on which they are reporting? 2) Do the news media discuss individual responsibility for weight more than the science on which they are reporting? 3) If either 1 or 2 is true, to what extent is this due to selective attention on the part of the news, e.g., to articles that lend themselves to drama or to a focus on individual blame? 4) What role do press releases play in determining which scientific articles receive media attention and how they are framed? Answering these questions sheds light not only on the respective roles played by news and science in constructing 'obesity' as a social problem but more generally on the mechanisms through which the news media disseminate medical science.

Data and Methods

To address these questions, we draw on a sample of scientific articles (N = 20) from two publications of the *Journal of the American Medical Association (JAMA)*, one of the two leading peer-reviewed medical journals. Our sample also includes relevant press releases (N = 8) and news reporting on those articles (N = 128). We analyzed and coded all of the research articles, preliminary communications, and editorials in the 1999 and 2003 special issues on obesity in the *JAMA*. *JAMA* special issues are newsworthy events in themselves that generate media attention. Comparing coverage of articles within a special issue has the methodological advantage of allowing us to hold constant other factors that affect media coverage, such as the moment in the news cycle and the prestige of the journal. Analysing two different issues, published four years apart, allows us to examine the effect of differences in news events (in this case the publication of each special issue) on news reporting.[2]

Findings: News Reporting on Obesity Science

Our analyses suggest that the news media take their cue from scientific studies when it comes to representing obesity as a crisis, but that they also throw 'fat on the fire' by using – more than the scientific studies on which they report – evocative words like 'epidemic' or 'war'. By referring to extreme examples as illustrative of the larger category of 'overweight' or 'obese', the news media magnify the perceived extent and scope of the 'obesity epidemic'. The news media are more likely than the science to ascribe individual blame for weight. Our matched sample allows us to show that these patterns are partly due to the reporters' selective attention to studies that lend themselves most readily to dramatization and a focus on individual blame. Press releases help explain both which articles the press report on and how those studies are framed.

Dramatization

Table 8.1 gives the proportion of scientific and news articles dramatizing obesity in various ways. The 1999 *JAMA* issue and news reporting on that issue overwhelmingly represented overweight and obesity as a crisis, at 70 per cent and 72 per cent, respectively. This framing was less prevalent in the 2003 special issue and news reporting on that issue, at 40 per cent and 34 per cent, respectively. It was not that the 2003 science and news articles countered claims that obesity was a crisis, but they were more likely to take them for granted. In both years, the

2 For more details on the data and methods, see: Saguy, A.C. & Almeling, R. (2008). Fat in the fire? Science, the news media, and the 'Obesity Epidemic'. *Sociological Forum, 23(1)*, 53–83.

Table 8.1 Proportion of scientific studies or news reports evoking specific frames

	1999 Science	1999 News	2003 Science	2003 News
DRAMA				
Crisis	0.70	0.72	0.40	0.34
Epidemic	0.20	0.49	0.20	0.31
War	0.00	0.46	0.00	0.27
Blurring weight categories	0.20	0.39	0.10	0.53
CAUSES				
Individual	0.40	0.72	0.40	0.98
Systemic	0.30	0.58	0.30	0.12
Genetic	0.1	0.1	0.2	0.03
SOLUTIONS				
Individual	0.80	0.74	0.90	0.81
Policy	0.50	0.35	0.20	0.17
Drugs	0.20	0.3	0.60	0.25
Surgery	0.00	0.01	0.20	0.08

science and news were equally likely to present obesity as a crisis. Twenty per cent of the articles in the 1999 special issue of *JAMA*, compared to 49 per cent of news reporting on that issue labelled obesity an epidemic. Two of the 10 scientific articles in the 2003 *JAMA* issue invoked the 'obesity epidemic', and 31 per cent of news coverage of this issue framed obesity as an epidemic. In neither year did the *JAMA* articles use war metaphors. Yet, 46 per cent of the 1999 news sample and 27 per cent of 2003 news reporting used war metaphors. A typical news report proclaimed that 'unless something is done to halt the trend, today's kids will grow up to be even heavier than their parents, already the fattest generation in history' (Ritter, 2003) and another reported that: 'There's a rapidly spreading epidemic afflicting all regions of the country, all ethnic and economic groups, and all ages … It's not SARS, West Nile virus, or Lyme disease. It's obesity' (Delude, 2003). Quoting a diabetes specialist, a 2003 news article declared obesity 'a time bomb' (Ritter, 2003).

While only one of the 2003 *JAMA* articles blurred the differences between weight categories, 53 per cent of news reports on this issue did. Most commonly, these articles took extreme examples in the context of a discussion about overweight or obesity. For instance, one article discussed a '285-pound' man and his '248-pound wife', 'a 100-pound 3-year-old girl', '417-pound 15-year-old boy', and children who 'had to be weighed on a loading dock scale' in a discussion of 'obesity', even though these individuals each have BMIs well above 40, a category which represents less than 5 per cent of the US population (Flegal et al., 2002). After reviewing these extreme cases, the article noted that '59% of Wisconsin adults already are either overweight or obese' (Fauber & Johnson, 2003b), giving the impression that extreme cases are more representative than they are.

As is shown in Table 8.1, the news media are most likely to air scientific debates when reporting on scientific studies that did so. Just as none of the scientific articles in either 1999 or 2003 alluded to any debate over whether weight *per se* was a meaningful indicator of health (obesity risk debate), neither did any of the press reports on these studies. Just as none of the *JAMA* articles in either the 1999 or 2003 special issues discussed the appropriate cut-off point between healthy and unhealthy weight, neither did news reports on these issues. All six news articles (or 9 per cent of the sample for that year) reporting on the 1999 study showing that physical fitness is a better predictor of health than weight (Wei et al., 1999) discussed the claim that one can be 'fat and fit'. For instance, an article in the *Philadelphia Inquirer* (McCullough, 1999) quotes one of the senior co-authors of the *JAMA* article saying: 'I think lack of activity is a far more important health risk than obesity'. Yet, none of the news reports used this research to critique any of the 1999 scientific studies, which made claims about body weight without statistically controlling for physical fitness. In 2003, two news stories (3 per cent of the sample for that year) discussed the 'fat and fit' argument even though none of the 2003 *JAMA* articles did. Both of these articles drew on other research or 'experts' to make this point.

Blame and Responsibility

News articles tended to attribute obesity to personal choices, especially those thought to reflect moral character, like choosing to be sedentary or making bad food choices. Table 8.1 gives the relative emphasis on individual, structural and genetic causes of obesity. In 1999, 72 per cent of news reports, compared to 40 per cent of the scientific articles, evoked individual contributors to weight. In 2003, 40 per cent of the science articles versus 98 per cent of reporting on that science stressed individual responsibility for weight. Among individual behaviours blamed for excess weight, the press was especially likely to focus on food choices and sedentary lifestyles. For instance, a Boston Globe article wrote that, like adults, children spend '*lazy* hours in front of the TV, which can be hazardous to both age groups' health and well-being' (Delude, 2003, emphasis added).

In many instances, the press used poetic license to paint a picture of sloth and gluttony. 'Americans are *gobbling down* more calories than ever, resulting in a 50 per cent increase in the nation's obesity rate', begins the first line of one typical news report (Torassa, 1999, emphasis added) on the 1999 study of the 'obesity epidemic' (Mokdad et al., 1999). Another news report on the 1999 special issue reports, 'Some 300,000 Americans die each year from *eating millions of cookies, hot dogs, potato chips* and other empty calories *during increasingly inactive lives*, according to another report also published in JAMA' (Hudson, 1999, emphasis added). That the scientific studies in question reported *no* data on the eating or exercise behaviours of their respondents did not prevent this or other press reports from speculating about individual excesses.

In the case of 'childhood obesity', parents, schools, and 'society' were blamed for 'buy[ing] our kids Oreos and Nintendos, eliminat[ing] gym classes to improve math scores, sell[ing] pizza at school fund-raisers, us[ing] the TV as a baby sitter and driv[ing] kids everywhere in minivans equipped with cup trays to hold milkshakes and Slurpees' (Ritter, 2003). Articles that pressure 'parents' to breastfeed as a way of preventing obesity and suggest that 'bottle-feeding parents might make their babies finish the bottle even when the kids feel full' (Ritter, 2003) more accurately target mothers. Discussions of childhood obesity were often racialized, as when an article asked whether 'greater acceptance of overweight and obesity among African American girls [...] contribute to the disproportionate percentages of obesity among minorities' and suggested that 'such sidestepping denies poor minority girls a principal – if sometimes unpleasant – psychological incentive to lose weight: that of social stigma' (Grossman, 2003). Among the entire news sample, news articles that mentioned the poor, blacks, or Latinos were statistically more likely – compared to those that did not mention these groups – to ascribe higher weights to poor food or exercise choices.

The 1999, but not 2003, news sample was also more likely to discuss systemic contributors to obesity. Specifically, in 1999, 58 per cent of the news reports, compared to 30 per cent of the *JAMA* articles, evoked social-structural contributors to obesity, including the food industry, the car culture, or urban planning. However, in 2003, 30 per cent of the *JAMA* articles, but only 12 per cent of news reporting on those articles, mentioned social-structural contributors. In both years, the news sources were more likely to mention social-structural contributors when discussing the poor, minorities, or children. One article quoted the coordinator of a food pantry who serves many poor families on Milwaukee's south side, who explained 'It's hard to eat healthy when you don't have the gas on or you're sleeping on the floor and you don't have a refrigerator' (Fauber & Johnson, 2003a). But most of the time, mentioning social structural factors did not serve to let individuals off the hook. Rather, industry and consumers were likely to be held jointly responsible, as in this article: 'They're pushing these super-sized foods at restaurants, and customers want value for their dollar ... Am I going to go to the restaurants where I get a 3-ounce burger for $3, or to the one where I get an 8-ounce burger for $3?' (Winiarski, 1999).

Only 10 per cent of articles in the 1999 *JAMA* issue and 10 per cent of news reporting on that issue mentioned genetic contributors to obesity. In 2003, only 3 per cent of the news mentioned genetic contributors to obesity, even though these were discussed by 20 per cent of the corresponding science sample. That the press hardly ever mentioned genetic contributors to weight, even when they were mentioned in the scientific journal on which they were reporting is striking and demonstrates the extent to which the news tends to attribute body size to individual volition. This, in turn, discredits claims that people should be protected from weight-based discrimination, since such protection is generally accorded to immutable traits, not chosen behaviour (see Saguy, 2013).

Finally, Table 8.1 gives the proportion of scientific and news articles that cite particular weight loss techniques or strategies, including individual changes to exercise or diet, any policy solutions, weight-loss drugs, or weight-loss surgery. Here, there is no clear pattern to the differences between science and media framing. Among solutions for perceived excess body weight, both scientific and news discussions were most likely to discuss individual behaviour modification, especially weight loss diets or exercise. In 1999, 80 per cent of the science sample and 74 per cent of the news sample mentioned people making changes to their diet or exercise patterns to lose weight. In 2003, these figures were 90 and 81 per cent for the science and news, respectively. Policy solutions were discussed considerably less often than individual behaviour modification. Nonetheless, in 1999, half of the science sample and 35 per cent of the news sample mentioned some sort of policy solution. These figures were 20 and 17 per cent for the 2003 science and news, respectively. Policy solutions were statistically more likely to be discussed, including favourably, when reporting on minorities or the poor, who may be perceived as lacking the resources to take action on their own. Likewise, discussion of public policy solutions were especially common when children were mentioned, consistent with the view of children as not fully capable of making their own choices.

Weight-loss drugs were discussed in 20 per cent of the 1999 science sample and 30 per cent of the 1999 news sample. In 2003, these figures were 60 per cent for the science and 25 per cent for the news samples.[3] News media discussions of weight-loss drugs usually highlighted their ineffectiveness, thus serving to further emphasize the importance of behaviour modification. For instance, one article quoted a Professor of Nutrition discussing weight-loss drugs as an elusive 'magic bullet' that distracts people from 'doing what they know they should do' (Hsu, 1999). Another article quoted the director of the Center for Science in the Public Interest, saying 'It may be that we enjoy our slothful, gluttonous lifestyle so much that we'll just remain overweight until we come up with a drug to cure it' (McCullough, 1999).

Weight-loss surgery was not mentioned in any of the 1999 science reports and in only one of the 1999 news reports. Twenty per cent of the 2003 science reports discussed weight-loss surgery, compared to 8 per cent of the 2003 news reports. Because weight-loss surgery does not repair faulty biological function (and in fact impairs some aspects of the proper functioning of the stomach such as assimilation of nutrients and vitamins), discussions of such surgery are quite consistent with blaming individuals for their weight, their inability to lose it, and their apparent need for drastic surgery to compensate for their personal failings. For instance,

3 This is because there were several articles in the 2003 *JAMA* issue that tested weight-loss drugs, but few news reports that discussed those particular articles, which speaks to the phenomenon of selective reporting discussed in the next section.

one article quoted a patient who said that she had surgery because she 'could not do it on [her] own' and a surgeon who blamed failed weight loss surgeries on patients who 'cheat' by 'eating certain types of food that limit their weight loss or cause them to gain back weight' (Fauber & Johnson, 2003b). Together, these findings suggest that, despite increased medicalization, body weight and eating are as moralized as ever.

Selective Reporting, Drama, and Individualizing

Our analyses suggest that selective reporting is an important mechanism through which the news sensationalizes its reporting on science. That is, journalists tend to cover articles that lend themselves to dramatization more than those that do not. For instance, in 1999, 43 news articles, over half of the total sample for that year, discussed 'The Spread of the Obesity Epidemic' (Mokdad et al., 1999). Moreover, as is shown in Table 8.2, those news articles that reported on this specific study were significantly more likely ($p < .000$) – compared to articles that did not discuss this study – to refer to obesity as an epidemic (67 vs. 19). A front-page *Milwaukee Journal Sentinel* article quoted the authors saying 'rarely do chronic conditions such as obesity spread with the speed and dispersion characteristics of a communicable disease epidemic' (Fauber, 1999).

The fact that press reporting in 2003 was more likely to blur the lines between different weight categories is also partly attributed to the disproportionate focus in 2003 on the one article that blurred the lines between different weight categories: 'Health related quality of life of severely obese children and adolescents' (Schwimmer et al., 2003). Although the title referred to 'severely obese' children and the abstract specified that the average BMI of participants was 34.7, both the abstract and article often referred simply to 'obese' children: 'Compared with healthy children and adolescents, obese children and adolescents reported significantly ($p < .001$) lower health-related [Quality of Life] QOL in all domains …'. This statement falsely implied that the research sample was representative of this larger group of youngsters. Similarly, almost all of the press reports on this study (15/16) suggested that this study pertained to obese or overweight children *in general*, rarely mentioning that the youngsters in the study were hospitalized and had serious health conditions. 'Obesity hurts kids' lifestyles like cancer', proclaimed one typical news headline (Fauber, 2003). In comparison, 31 per cent of news articles that did not explicitly mention the quality-of-life article blurred the lines between weight categories, a still sizable but much smaller proportion.

While selective reporting can help shed light on why the press was more likely than the science on which it was reporting to represent obesity as an epidemic and to blur weight categories, it does not seem to explain the greater tendency of the press in 1999 or 2003 to use war metaphors like 'battle' or 'time bomb'. This language was not significantly more likely, for either given year, to appear in news articles that reported on the 1999 'obesity epidemic' article, the 1999

Table 8.2 News framing by scientific article covered

	Mentioned study	Do not mention study	Difference
Epidemic	0.67	0.19	0.48***
Blurring categories	0.94	0.31	0.63**
Individual blame	0.88	0.64	0.24*

Note: The scientific studies mentioned were Mokdad et al., Schwimmer et al. and Allison et al. for epidemic, blurring the weight categories, and individual blame, respectively; *** $p < .000$, ** $p < .001$, * $p < .05$; Based on a Fisher's Exact Test (two-sided).

'annual deaths' article, the 2003 'low-carb' article (Bravata et al., 2003), or the 2003 'Quality of Life' article (Schwimmer et al., 2003). This suggests that this particular difference is driven by general media routines that favour 'war' imagery rather than by selective reporting. Use of such metaphors in press releases – a topic we discuss below – may also foster their prevalence in the news.

Why is the press more likely to focus on individual contributors to obesity than are the scientific studies on which they are reporting? Because almost all of the press reports in 2003 blamed weight on individual factors, we have virtually no variance to explain for this year. In 1999, over 70 per cent of press reports discussed individual contributors to weight, but we can still find variation among these 69 news articles. Twenty-four of these articles reported on Allison et al's (1999) 'Annual deaths attributable to obesity in the United States'. Using methodology originally formulated to calculate 'tobacco deaths', Allison et al. assumed that 'obesity-attributable deaths' were avoidable and due to unhealthy individual choices. The disproportionate attention given to this article by the media seems to have contributed to the framing of weight as a product of individual choices or behaviours. Articles that mentioned the 'annual deaths' study were significantly more likely than articles that did not mention this study ($p < 0.05$) to suggest that weight is determined by individual behaviour. Eighty-eight per cent of press reports on this scientific study invoked individual contributors to weight, compared to 64 per cent of articles that did not explicitly discuss this study.

The Role of Press Releases

We find some evidence that press releases also shape which research receives the most media attention and how research is framed. Press releases offer pre-packaged news that can easily be turned into copy by time-pressed journalists. In 1999, coverage in the *JAMA* or CDC press release was an excellent predictor of news coverage. The four studies that were most prominently featured in the 1999 *JAMA* press release (Mokdad et al., 1999; Koplan and Dietz, 1999; Allison et al., 1999; Heymsfield et al., 1999) were the same ones that received the most media attention, although not in this precise order. In 2003, coverage by press releases was a less reliable predictor of news coverage than in 1999.

Moreover, the way in which press releases present science seems to shape news framing. In 1999, when the news reports were more likely than the *JAMA* articles to use war metaphors, refer to obesity as an epidemic, or to stress individual contributors towards obesity, the official *JAMA* press release also included all three of those frames. In 2003, when the press was more likely than the *JAMA* articles to use war metaphors, stress individual contributors towards obesity, and blur the lines between different weight categories, the official *JAMA* press release included the first two of these three frames. This underscores the important intermediary role that press releases have in framing news reports. The 2003 official *JAMA* press release, which did not mention the quality of life article (Schwimmer et al., 2003), did not blur the lines between weight categories. However, a separate press release that was released by the University of California – San Diego, where the lead author was employed, to promote this particular article did blur the lines between weight categories.

Conclusion

In this chapter, we exploit a unique sample of: 1) scientific articles on weight and health; 2) press releases on those studies; and 3) news reports on those same studies to shed new light on how the news media filter and translate scientific information to the lay public. We found some evidence that news media enflamed the issue, while emphasizing individual blame. Compared to the science on which they were reporting, the news media used more evocative metaphors and language to discuss this putative crisis. The use of epidemic metaphors was largely attributable to the disproportionate media attention received by one of 10 scientific articles in the special issue. Selective reporting also partially explained the news media's greater tendency to blame individuals for their weight. Our findings further suggest that press releases foster dramatization.

This study has shown how scientific and news media discussions of weight assess blame and responsibility for body weight. We found that both science and news blame individual choices for excess weight more than social structural or genetic factors, and that the news further accentuates the focus on individual blame. Individual solutions are even more likely to be invoked, compared to policy or biological solutions. Discussing certain groups – including children, African-Americans, Latinos, or the poor – increases the likelihood of blaming individuals (or their parents) or social-structural factors and of discussing policy solutions. In that women are usually held responsible as parents, parental blame is implicitly targeted at women.

These findings support the contention that scientists work as 'parajournalists' (Schudson, 2003), writing up their studies – especially the abstract – with journalists in mind. They then frame their research via press releases and interviews with journalists. A reward structure in which, all things being equal, alarmist studies are more likely to be covered in the media may make scientists even more prone to presenting their findings in the most dramatic light possible.

Do journalists, in turn, function as 'parascientists'? No, if the definition of a parascientist involves independently evaluating research studies. However, journalists can raise questions about research by citing sceptical 'experts' or shape public understandings of the scientific field by featuring some research while ignoring others. We found ample evidence that the news media report more on some studies than others, but little evidence of the news media expressing scepticism of the research on which they were reporting, either directly or via new sources.

In that how public issues are framed shapes private and public action, the patterns that we have documented have far-reaching social implications. As obesity is widely accepted as a dire health risk, we may become more tolerant of health risks associated with weight loss treatments, enact public policies designed to promote weight loss on a population level, and prioritize funding for obesity research over competing causes. Indeed, in recent years, funds for tobacco research have declined as funds for obesity research climb (Saguy, 2006). On the other hand, news reports of 'obesity' as a public health crisis may make competing frames of 'fat' as a neutral and positive form of biological diversity more difficult to promote. Not only are such news reports likely to reinforce the stigma of fat bodies as diseased bodies, but in that they tend to liken fatness to a health *behaviour*, they undermine the claim that weight is an immutable trait. This presents a challenge for proponents of weight-based anti-discrimination laws. Gay rights activists have faced similar resistance from people who regard sexual 'preference' as a choice or lifestyle. Arguments about the genetic basis of homosexuality have been politically contested because it is widely perceived as a prerequisite for gaining civil rights for gays and lesbians.

In sum, science reporting informs lay understandings of health and risk, policy priorities, blame and responsibility, and normative understandings of acceptable and desirable bodies. We invite others to join us in studying public discussions of body weight and their implications for moral hierarchies and social control.

References

Allison, D.B., Fontaine, K.R., Mansen, J.E., et al. (1999). Annual deaths attributable to obesity in the United States. *JAMA*, *282(16)*, 1530–1538.

Associated Press. (2006). Surgeon General: Obesity epidemic will dwarf terrorism threat. *Health SciTech*, March 2.

Bennett, W.L. (1983). *News: The politics of illusion.* New York: Longman.

Bish, C.L., Blanck, H.M., Serdula, M.K., et al. (2005). Diet and physical activity behaviors among Americans trying to lose weight: 2000 behavioral risk factor surveillance system. *Obesity Research*, *13*, 596–607.

Bordo, S. (1993). *Unbearable weight: Feminism, western culture, and the body.* Berkeley: University of California Press.
Bravata, D.M., Sanders, L., Huang, J., et al. (2003). Efficacy and safety of low-carbohydrate diets: A systematic review. *JAMA, 289(14)*, 1837–1850.
Brownell, K. & Horgen, K.B. (2003). *Food fight: The inside story of the food industry, America's obesity crisis, and what we can do about it.* McGraw-Hill.
Calasanti, T.M. & Slevin, K.F. (2001). *Gender, social inequalities, and aging.* Lanham, MD: Alta Mira Press.
Campos, P. (2004). *The obesity myth.* New York : Gotham Books.
Campos, P., Saguy, A., Ernsberger, P., et al. (2006). The epidemiology of overweight and obesity: Public health crisis or moral panic? *International Journal of Epidemiology, 35(1)*, 55–60.
Carlsson, M.E. (2000). Cancer patients seeking information from sources outside the health care system. *Supportive Care in Cancer, 8(6)*, 453–457.
Chernin, K. (1995). *The hungry self: Women, eating, and identity.* New York: HarperCollins.
Clarke, J.N. & Everest, M.M. (2006). Cancer in the mass print media: Fear, uncertainty and the medical model. *Social Science and Medicine, 62*, 2591–2600.
Conrad, P. & Schneider, J.W. (1992). *Deviance and medicalization: From badness to sickness*. Philadelphia, PA: Temple University Press.
Conrad, P. & Markens, S. (2001). Constructing the 'gay gene' in the news: Optimism and skepticism in the US and British press. *Health, 5(3)*, 373–400.
Cooper, C. (1998). *Fat and proud: The politics of size*. London: Women's Press.
Crawford, R. (1980). Healthism and the medicalization of everyday life. *International Journal of Health Services, 10*, 365–388.
Dalton, S. (2004). *Our overweight children: What parents, schools, and communities can do to control the fatness epidemic*. Berkeley: University of California Press.
Darnton, R. (1975). Writing news and telling stories. *Daedalus, 104*, 175–194.
Delude, C.M. (2003). Time to take a vacation from television as school ends, keep kids healthy by limiting TV time. *The Boston Globe* (Boston, MA), HEALTH SCIENCE, June 10, C14.
Edgley, C. & Brissett, D. (1990). Health Nazis and the cult of the perfect body: Some polemic observations. *Symbolic Interaction, 13(2)*, 257–279.
Entman, R.M. (1993). Framing: Toward clarification of a fractured paradigm. *Journal of Communication, 43(4)*, 51–58.
Epstein, S. (1996). *Impure science: AIDS.* Berkeley: University of California Press.
Ericson, R.V., Baranek, P.M. & Chan, J.B.C. (1989). *Negotiating control: A study of news sources*. Toronto, Canada: University of Toronto Press.
Ernsberger, P. & Haskew, P. (1987). *Rethinking obesity: An alternative view of its health implications*. New York: Human Sciences Press.
Fauber, J. (1999). Obesity 'epidemic' sweeping nation: Studies show sharp increase in percentage of dangerously overweight adults in U.S. *Milwaukee Journal Sentinel* (Milwaukee, Wisconsin), News, 27 October, p. 1.

Fauber, J. (2003). Obesity hurts kids' lifestyles like cancer; obesity hurts kids' lifestyles like cancer, study finds. *Milwaukee Journal Sentinel* (Milwaukee, Wisconsin), News, 9 April, p. 01A.

Fauber, J. & Johnson, M. (2003a). Super-size problem; Americans' struggle with obesity takes breathtaking toll. *Milwaukee Journal Sentinel* (Milwaukee, Wisconsin), News, 6 July, p. 01A.

Fauber, J. & Johnson, M. (2003b). Losing weight; HEAVY BURDEN; THE OBESITY EPIDEMIC. *Milwaukee Journal Sentinel*, NEWS, 8 July, p. 01A.

Flegal, K.M., Carroll, M.D., Ogden, C.L. & Johnson, C.L. (2002). Prevalence and trends in obesity among US adults, 1999–2000. *JAMA, 288(14)*, 1723–1727.

Flegal, K.M., Graubard, B.I., Williamson, D.F. & Gail, M.H. (2005). Excess deaths associated with underweight, overweight, and obesity. *JAMA, 293(15)*, 1861–1867.

Fontanarosa, P.B. (1999). Patients, physicians, and weight control. *JAMA, 282(16)*, 1581–1582.

Fraser, L. (1998). *Losing it: False hopes and fat profits in the diet industry*. New York: Penguin Putnam Inc.

Gaesser, G.A. (1996). *Big fat lies: The truth about your weight and your health*. New York: Fawcett Columbine.

Gamson, W. (1992). *Talking politics*. Cambridge: Cambridge University Press.

Gans, H. (1979). *Deciding what's news*. New York: Pantheon.

Gieryn, T.F. & Figert, A.E. (1990). Ingredients for a theory of science in society: O-rings, ice water, C-clamp, Richard Feynman, and the press. In S.E. Cozzens & T.F. Gieryn (eds), *Theories of science in society* (pp. 67–97). Bloomington, IN: Indiana University Press.

Goffman, E. (1963). *Stigma: Notes on the management of a spoiled identity*. New York: Prentice-Hall.

Gusfield, J.R. (1981). *The culture of public problems: Drinking-driving and the symbolic order*. Chicago: University of Chicago Press.

Hesse-Biber, S. (1996). *Am I thin enough yet?: The cult of thinness and the commericialization of identity*. New York: Oxford University Press.

Heymsfield, S.B., Greenberg. A.S., Fujioka, K., et al. (1999). Recombinant leptin for weight loss in obese and lean adults: A randomized, controlled, dose-escalation trial. *JAMA, 282(16)*, 1568–1575.

Hsu, K. (1999). As US obesity rises, scientists see health crisis. *The Boston Globe*, NATIONAL/FOREIGN, 27 October, p. A3.

Hudson, M. (1999). America is fat, getting fatter; nearly 1 in 5 obese; results can be fatal. *Times-Picayune*, National, 27 October, p. A1.

Kuczmarski, R.J., Flegal, K.M., Campbell, S.M. & Johnson, C.L. (1994). Increasing prevalence of overweight among US adults: The National Health and Nutrition Examination Surveys, 1960 to 1991. *JAMA, 272*, 205–211.

Kwan, S. (2009). Framing the fat body: Contested meanings between government, activists, and industry. *Sociological Inquiry, 79*, 25–50.

Lawrence, R.G. (2003). Framing obesity: The evolution of news discourse on a public health issue. *Press/Politics, 9(3)*, 56–75.
LeBesco, K. (2004). The queerness of fat. In *Revolting bodies? The struggle to redefine fat identity* (pp. 85–97). Boston: University of Massachusetts Press.
Linn, S. (2004). *Consuming kids: The hostile takeover of childhood.* New York: New Press.
Lovric, L. (2005). Child obesity a form of abuse. *Winnipeg Sun*, 6 June.
Lupton, D. (1995). *The imperative of health: Public health and the regulated body*. London: Sage Publications.
Lyman, S.M. (1989). *The seven deadly sins: Society and evil.* Dix Hills, NY: General Hall, Inc.
McCullough, M. (1999). Time for new approaches to weight loss. *The Philadelphia Inquirer*, DOMESTIC NEWS, 27 October.
McKenna, M.A.J. (1999). Georgians' weight problem is growing fast, study says. *The Atlanta Journal and Constitution* (Atlanta, GA), News, 27 October, p. 1A.
Millman, M. (1980). *Such a pretty face: Being fat in America.* New York, NY: W.W. Norton & Company.
Mokdad, A.H., Marks, J.S., Stroup, D.F. & Gerberding, J.L. (2004). Actual causes of death in the United States, 2000. *JAMA, 291(10)*, 1238–1245.
Mokdad, A.H., Serdula, M.K., Dietz, W.H., et al. (1999). The spread of the obesity epidemic in the United States, 1991–1998. *JAMA, 282(16)*, 1519–1522.
Moyniham, R. (2006). Expanding definitions of obesity may harm children. *British Medical Journal, 332*, 1412.
Nelkin, D. (1987). *Selling science: How the press covers science and technology.* Freeman.
Nestle, M. (2002). *Food politics: How the food industry influences nutrition and health.* Berkeley: University of California Press.
Nichter, M. (2000). *Fat talk: What girls and their parents say about dieting.* Cambridge, MA: Harvard University Press.
Oliver, J.E. (2005). *Fat politics: The real story behind America's obesity epidemic.* New York: Oxford University Press.
Oliver, J.E. (2006). The politics of pathology: How obesity became an epidemic disease. *Perspectives in Biology and Medicine, 49(4)*, 611–627.
Ritter, J. (2003). Kids on front lines of obesity war. *Chicago Sun-Times*, 1 July, p. 8.
Saguy, A. (2006). Are Americans too fat? Conversation with Stanton Glantz. *Contexts, 5(2)*, 11–13.
Saguy, A.C. (2013). *What's wrong with fat?* New York: Oxford University Press.
Saguy, A.C. & Riley, K.W. (2005). Weighing both sides: Morality, mortality and framing contests over obesity. *Journal of Health Politics, Policy, and Law, 30(5)*, 869–921.
Santry, H.P., Gillen, D.L. & Lauderdale, D.S. (2005). Trends in bariatric surgical procedures. *JAMA, 294(15)*, 1909–1917.

Schlesinger, M. (2002). A loss of faith: The sources of reduced political legitimacy for the American medical profession. *The Milbank Quarterly, 80(2)*, 185–235.
Schoenfielder, L. & Wieser, B. (1983). *Shadow on a tightrope: Writings by women on fat oppression.* Iowa City: Aunt Lute Book Company.
Schudson, M. (2003). *The sociology of the news.* New York: W.W. Norton & Company.
Schwimmer, J.B., Burwinkle, T.M. & Varni, J.W. (2003). Health-related quality of life of severely obese children and adolescents. *JAMA, 289(14)*, 1813–1819.
Snow, D. & Benford, R.D. (1988). Ideology, frame resonance and participant mobilization. *International Social Movement Research, 1*, 197–217.
Sobal, J. (1995). The medicalization and demedicalization of obesity. In D. Maurer & J. Sobal (eds), *Eating agendas* (pp. 67–90). New York: Aldine de Gruyter.
Spector, M. & Kitsuse, J.I. (1977). *Constructing social problems.* Menlo Park, CA: Cummings Publishing Company, Inc.
Stein, H.F. (1982a). 'Health' and 'wellness' and euphemism: The cultural context of insidious draconian health policy, *Continuing Education* (March), 33–44.
Stein, H.F. (1982b). Wellness as illusion. *Delaware Medical Journal, 54(11)*, 637–641.
Tarrow, S. (1992). Mentalities, political cultures, and collective action frames: Constructing meanings through action. In A.D. Morris & C.M. Mueller (eds), *Frontiers in social movement theory* (pp. 174–202). New Haven and London: Yale University Press.
Tartamella, L., Herscher, E. & Woolston, C. (2005). *Generation extra large: Rescuing our children from the epidemic of obesity.* New York: Basic Books.
Tesh, S.N. (1988). *Hidden arguments: Political ideology and disease prevention policy.* New Brunswick, NJ: Rutgers University Press.
Thompson, B.W. (1994). *A hunger so wide and so deep: A multiracial view of women's eating problems.* Minneapolis: University of Minnesota Press.
Torassa, U.P. (1999). Americans keep packing on the pounds. *San Francisco Examiner*, National, 27 October, p. 1A.
Tuchman, G. (1978). *Making news: A study in the construction of reality.* New York: Free Press.
Wann, M. (1999). *FAT! SO?: Because you don't have to apologize for your size.* Berkeley: Ten Speed Press.
Wei, M., Kampert, J.B., Barlow, C.E., et al. (1999). Relationship between low cardiorespiratory fitness and mortality in normal-weight, overweight, and obese men. *JAMA, 282*, 1547–1553.
Winiarski, K. (1999). Over half of South Carolina adults are overweight, Health Department. *The State*, 23 November.
Wolf, N. (1991). *The beauty myth: How images of beauty are used against women.* New York: William Morrow and Company, Inc.

Chapter 9

Obesity, Government and the Media

Stanley Ulijaszek

The relationship between government and media is one of constant negotiation, influenced by political ideologies, constituencies and markets. News media help to set public and policy agendas, are involved in the process of defining hazards as risks, and influence people's health behaviours (Bonfiglioli et al., 2011). The news media draw attention to, and indeed frame, particular issues as problems that might be of interest or entertainment value to their reading and viewing audiences, with heavy coverage often raising the profile of these issues on public policy agendas (Entman, 1993). In the battles for hearts and minds waged by a range of interest groups (including policy-makers, political lobbies, and citizen advocates), the media have great power in telling the public what to think about, if not what they should think. Developed by McCombs and Shaw (1972) during the 1968 United States presidential election, agenda-setting theory has shown repeatedly that public concern and policy attention rise and fall in response to shifts in media coverage rather than changes in the size of the problem itself (Boyce, 2007). In the United Kingdom (UK), obesity became an issue of concern for health from the 1970s, and of concern for economists since the 1980s. Governmental press offices have been increasingly communicating policies and the documents that support their formation to the news media (including newspapers, television, and most recently online news sources), in attempts to influence public understanding and individual behaviour around obesity and its causation.

The logic of news reporting involves disseminating what is novel, what affects the public, and whether social institutions are effective in addressing public challenges. News media take a critical stance towards authority of any kind, including that of medical science (Picard & Yeo, 2011). Policy makers face a range of challenges when seeking to disseminate anti-obesity messages via the news media. While policy and policy-related documents can come from many sources, governmental sources may come under critical media scrutiny because of the power that the originators of these documents have.

In both the United States (US) and the UK, the media operate within market-liberal frameworks, which draw heavily upon concepts of individualism and the rationality of the market in framing problem-solving. In the US, the reporting of obesity by news media is usually framed as a crisis, caused by individual lack of control, to be solved by individuals taking control (of their eating, their lifestyles, and their behaviours) (Saguy & Almeling, this volume). Concepts of systemic causation involving multiple actors, including political and sociostructural elements, receive much less attention, as do policy solutions. However, over the past decade, a time when obesity rates have continued to rise in most age and gender groups, the UK has seen shifts in the framing of obesity-related problems by experts and policy-makers, with individual-centred messages being increasingly tempered or even supplanted by more ecological approaches.

This chapter will examine the ways in which UK governmental obesity policy and framework documents have been interpreted and reported by the news media across the past 11 years. Until mid-2010, the UK was under Labour administration, in a marketized form of social democracy. From May 2010 onward, the UK has been governed by a Conservative-led Liberal Democrat coalition, which in largest part has favoured more marketized solutions to problems than the Labour government had. Across this period, the scientific and medical discourse about obesity has seen shifts from personal to social responsibility and back to personal responsibility again. This was also a period in which policy thinking about obesity briefly shifted from solutions based on individual responsibility to ones that encompassed complexity of causation and multiply-coordinated actions, before quickly returning to solutions based on individual responsibility again.

Types of Obesity Policy

Obesity is complex and many frameworks are used to try to explain it, including those of genetics, physiology, psychology, economics, anthropology, and sociology (Ulijaszek, 2008). Each framework offers different possibilities for action by policy makers, but the plurality of interpretations has so far led to confusion, caution and often inaction (Lang & Rayner, 2007). There are competing ideas of what the most important factors are in the production of population obesity (Ulijaszek, 2008), which complicates the policy making process. Across the industrialized world, a wide range of analyses and policy solutions has been developed and proffered, the increasing sophistication of different policy positions adding to the complexity of policy development and roll-out (Lang & Rayner, 2007).

Food governance issues further complicate obesity policy formulation and implementation. For example, food policy can be influenced by global, European, national, regional, and local factors. Food subsidies from the European Union Common Agricultural Policy promote the production of some foods over others, and this can influence shopping patterns through price. Such upstream factors are important when policy is shaped at national, regional and local levels (Musingarimi, 2008). Ideological issues, such as the restriction of personal choices and freedoms in food and lifestyle, also effect policy, as well as public perception of what type of issue obesity is, and why people should be concerned. The issue of obesity has potential to be compelling to the public through a number of lenses: health and well-being; appearance and attractiveness; stigma and discrimination; job aspiration and satisfaction; income and inequality; status; personal responsibility; personal freedom; state intervention; and childhood protection.

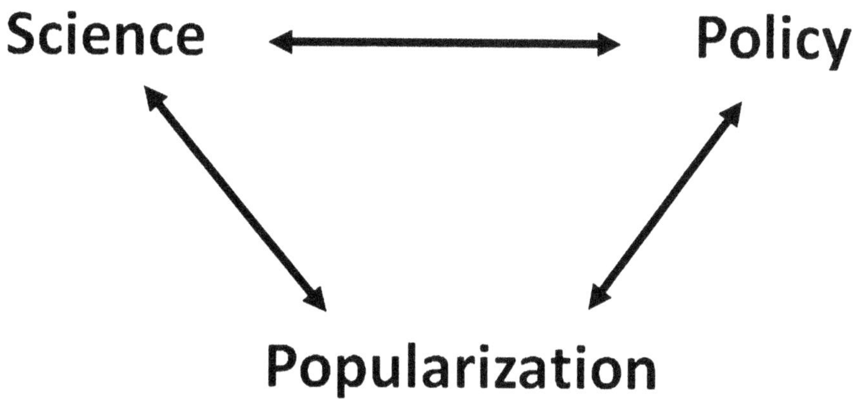

Figure 9.1 Agenda setting for obesity policy

The news media are able to frame how the public thinks about obesity: if media coverage of obesity is predominantly of health and well-being, public concern in this domain might follow, and policy might also follow, in turn. Alternatively, if the news media focus were on the economic costs of obesity, this would be convergent with governmental concerns about the high obesity-related health care costs, and of the extent to which obesity-related illness resulted in lost economic productivity. If, however, news media were concerned with the relationships between obesity, income and inequality, then this might increase scrutiny on government with regard to policy and social inequality.

There is an uneasy relationship between the news media and government with respect to agenda setting of policy more generally (Figure 9.1). News media can influence government through continual and persistent shaping of public awareness. The scope for political ideology to shape public awareness for managing and reducing obesity prevalence therefore depends on the extent to which the media are *on-message* with the ideas and policies of the dominant political party. This is unstable because the news media depend on public consumption for their financial success. The news media thrive on reporting of novelty, but this is often at odds with the reality that important new observations are rare. And the news media's critical stance with respect to institutions other than themselves sits uneasily with government.

There is a large number of sources from which obesity policy can emanate in the UK, and this adds to the cacophony of obesity policy formation. Makers of obesity and obesity-related policy are diverse, including governmental and non-governmental organizations. The Association for the Study of Obesity (2011) published a briefing paper which lists key policy documents, strategies and recommendations on obesity in the UK between 2000 and 2010 (Table 9.1). It lists eight key reports, 12 key strategy documents, four public service agreements, and 10 National Institute for Health and Clinical Excellence (NICE) sets of

Table 9.1 Key *policy* documents, strategies and recommendations on *obesity* in the UK between 2000 and 2010 (Association for the Study of Obesity 2011)

Key reports
National Audit Office (2001) Tackling obesity in England
Annual report of the Chief Medical Officer 2002
Chief Medical Officer (2004) At least five a week: evidence on the impact of physical activity and its relationship to health
House of Commons Health Select Committee report on Obesity 2004
Wanless (2004) Securing good health for the whole population
National Audit Office (2006) Tackling obesity: first steps
Foresight (2007) Tackling obesities: future choices
Marmot (2010) Fair society, healthy lives: a strategic review of health inequalities in England
Key strategy documents
Cancer Plan (2000)
National Service Framework for Coronary Heart Disease (2000)
National Service Framework for Diabetes (2001)
Tackling health inequalities – a programme for action (2003)
Department for Children Schools and Families (2003) Every child matters (delivered through the Children's Plan (2007), including Healthy Lives, Brighter Futures strategy and the Play Strategy
Choosing Health: White Paper 2004
Choosing Activity: a physical activity action plan (2005)
Choosing a better diet (2005)
National service framework for children, young people and maternity services (2004)
Healthy Weight, Healthy Lives: a cross government strategy (2008)
Be active be healthy: a plan for getting the nation moving (Department of Health 2009)
Food 2030 (2010) Defra
Public Service Agreements, relevant to obesity and obesity-related factors 2008–11
PSA 12: Improve the health and well-being of children and young people Breastfeeding at six to eight weeks Take up of school lunches Childhood obesity
PSA 21: Build more cohesive, empowered and active communities Percentage of people who feel that they belong to their neighbourhood
PSA 22: Deliver a successful Olympic games Children and young people's participation in sport
PSA 23: Make communities safer Percentage of people perceiving anti-social behaviour as a problem

clinical guidance and public health guidance notes that include obesity. The latter include the following documents: Four commonly used methods to increase physical activity (2006); Maternal and child nutrition (2008); Physical activity and the environment (2008); Promoting physical activity in the workplace (2008);

Table 9.2 Arm's-length bodies (non-governmental organizations usually sponsored by government) sponsored by the Department of Health and other non-governmental organizations producing obesity and obesity-related policy documents between 2000 and 2010

Arms-length bodies
Cycling England
Commission for Architecture and the Built Environment
Food Standards Agency (Responsibility for nutrition moved to DH in 2010)
Care Quality Commission (formerly the Healthcare Commission)
Local Government Improvement and Development [Formerly IDeA]
National Institute for Health and Clinical Excellence
Natural England
Ofcom
Ofsted
School Food Trust
Sport England
Sustainable Development Commission
Non-governmental organizations
Royal College of Obstetricians and Gynaecologists
Royal College of Paediatrics and Child Health
Faculty of Public Health
British Dietetic Association
Diabetes UK
Association of Chief Executives of Voluntary Organisations
Caroline Walker Trust
National Heart Forum
National Obesity Forum
Sustrans

Promoting physical activity for children and young people (2009); Prevention of cardiovascular disease (2010); Alcohol-use disorders – preventing harmful drinking (2010); Weight management before, during and after pregnancy (2010); and Preventing type 2 diabetes: population and community level interventions in high risk groups and the general population (2011). They also note that guidance and recommendation documents have been produced by 12 arm's-length bodies sponsored by the Department of Health (including NICE) and 10 non-government organizations across this period (Table 9.2). Most arm's-length bodies either deliver public services or provide specialist advice to Government.

This wide range of sources has given the news media great scope for identifying novelty in thinking about anti-obesity policy and a broad menu of options with which to frame the obesity problem. Clearly, not all obesity or obesity-related policy is, or can be, reported, and it is difficult to relate the publication of reports from most organizations to particular news items. For this reason, the relationship between what is published and released to the news media and what is published by the news media is examined here in relation to a small number of higher-profile cases. Each is a governmental publication that carried weight in the formation of UK anti-obesity policy. They are as follows: the National Audit Office's 'Tackling Obesity in England' (2001); 'The House of Commons Health Select Committee Report on Obesity' (2004); 'Foresight: Tackling Obesities: Future Choices' (2007); and 'Healthy lives, Healthy People – A Call to Action on Obesity in England' (2010). Documents from arms-length bodies and non-governmental organizations are not considered because they represent a diversity of interests from institutions which hold variable influence on policy-making, from low to high, and whose policy documents often do not gain so much media attention.

National Audit Office (2001): 'Tackling Obesity in England'

The National Audit Office's (2001) publication 'Tackling Obesity in England' reported on the tripling of obesity rates in England over the past 20 years. It also reported on population obesity's purported costs to the National Health Service (NHS), as well as to the wider economy, because of lower productivity and lost output. The report emphasized the need for an evidence-based approach to obesity to enable the NHS to adopt a more consistent strategy to its management. It went on to recommend the implementation of nutrition initiatives in the NHS, including the Five-a-Day fruits and vegetables campaign, the Food in Schools programme, the promotion and support of infant feeding, and welfare food programmes, as well as the development of a cross-government strategy for obesity control and prevention.

Northrop (n.d.) carried out a content analysis of articles appearing in *The Sun*, *Daily Mail* and *The Guardian* newspapers at the time of the publication of this report . All three newspapers used headlines that emphasized: 1) factual information from the report, 2) obesity as an issue of national concern; and 3) childhood obesity. Other headlines focused on individual experiences, usually from people who had been obese and had successfully dieted. One celebrity dieter also featured in a headline in the *Daily Mail* newspaper. Themes raised in the articles included risk, blame and responsibility. All three newspapers presented factual information from research on childhood obesity and The National Audit Committee's report. They included the economic cost and the possible causes for the increase in obesity and overweight in Britain.

In all cases, expert opinion was sought and comments given from either medical doctors, nutritionists, or representatives of the Department of Health. An article published in *The Guardian* on 15 February 2001 (Meikle, 2001) provides an example of this use of expert opinion. James Robertson, director of health value for money at the National Audit Office, was quoted as saying: 'It is a mistake to say there is a problem which cannot be tackled. There need not be a counsel of desperation. We are not seeking a nanny state'. Suzi Leather, deputy chairman of the Food Standards Agency, was quoted as saying: 'We won't fight flab with only willpower. Consumers also need to be armed with information about the nutritional content of food. Improved labelling could do a great deal to help'. At a time when the UK government was trying to reduce welfare expenditures, the experts cited identified individual responsibility as the key to curbing the rising rates of obesity: the government's role was to provide nutritional information, but it was the citizens' responsibility to integrate this information into their own lives. These newspapers also turned to the food industry, which was characterized as 'cooperating with government and health bodies in attempting to reduce levels of ingredients such as salt in the public's diet and providing lifestyle advice, but remaining suspicious of state dictation' (Meikle, 2001).

In all three newspapers, journalistic advice was given about how further increases in obesity rates might be mitigated. Journalists emphasized lifestyle factors, nutrition and individual behaviour as being key to explaining the rise in obesity rates in the UK. Lifestyle factors included the increased use of cars, television and computer games, and the disconnection between ancestral (non-obesogenic) hunter-gatherer lifestyles and food seasonality, and present-day environments that contribute to obesity (Northrop, n.d.). With respect to nutrition, journalists emphasized the problems of consuming foods that were categorized as being fatty, junk, or convenient. They were also concerned with the sponsorship of schools by food companies, and the use of food to pacify very young children. Individual behaviour did not feature in news reports but in newspaper sections that dealt with health and diet. Articles that reported on individuals' personal experiences were used either as supporting material for the main story concerning the National Audit Office report, or to promote particular diets highlighted on the health pages. The novelty of this report lay in revealing a tripling of obesity rates, while promising that governmental institutions were undertaking the public challenge of controlling obesity, even if it were yet not under control. The breadth of response to the report by the media reflects the absence of clear thinking about the obesity problem in the UK at that time, and the sense that obesity rates had risen in the absence of effective governmental interventions.

House of Commons Health Select Committee Report on Obesity 2004

While the National Audit Office (2001) publication 'Tackling Obesity in England' stated the importance of obesity as an ever-rising health problem, and suggested the NHS should implement a range of initiatives to address it, the House of Commons Health Select Committee report on Obesity (2004) attempted to stimulate further interest in obesity by sensationalizing parts of the report. The likely influence of the report in shaping discourse, practice and dominant knowledge about obesity in both policy and popular media contexts in the UK was recognized by its authors, when they stated that 'this inquiry has contributed to the huge publicity that the subject of obesity has prompted over the last year or two' (House of Commons, 2004). In addition to highlighting the rapidly rising rates of obesity, its potential health consequences, and the need to increase physical activity and focus on preventing obesity in children, it had passages that starkly linked obesity to premature death. For example:

> Should the gloomier scenarios relating to obesity turn out to be true, the sight of amputees will become much more familiar in the streets of Britain. There will be many more blind people. There will be huge demand for kidney dialysis. The positive trends of recent decades in combating heart disease, partly the consequence of the decline in smoking, will be reversed. Indeed, this will be the first generation where children die before their parents as a consequence of childhood obesity.

It also attempted to individualize obesity, perhaps taking a note from journalistic practice, in reporting the obesity-related death of a 3-year-old child. In its second paragraph it stated:

> Dr Sheila McKenzie, a consultant at the Royal London Hospital which recently opened an obesity service for children, offered a powerful insight into the crisis posed to the nation's health. Despite only being in existence for three years, her service had an eleven-month waiting list. Over the last two years, she had witnessed a child of three dying from heart failure where extreme obesity was a contributory factor. Four of the children in the care of her unit were being managed at home with non-invasive ventilatory assistance for sleep apnoea: as she put it, "in other words, they are choking on their own fat".

This strategy back-fired, however. On the afternoon of the 26th May, 2004, the day before the release of the House of Commons Health Select Committee Report on Obesity (HCHSCRO) and its attendant press conference,

> Radio 4's Today programme ... had been leaked a story that MPs would report the case of an obese child who died of heart failure. By the evening, the media was saying that the report was critical of both the government and the food industry, and called for the banning of food advertising aimed at children. The following morning, national newspapers carried headlines like "Obesity kills child of 3". (Sanders, 2004: 1503)

Another prominent headline, which appeared in the *Daily Express*, read: 'Child, 3, dies from being too fat' (Wheldon, 2004). As Sanders (2004) notes, other headlines included: 'Choking our children on their fat' and 'Food will carry fat warning'. Many articles characterized this event as the result of child abuse.

Over a week later, journalists had identified sources that spoke to the child's extreme obesity as having been an outcome of 'a serious genetic defect', and the fact that 'the child had died before treatment could be offered' (Sanders, 2004). The misrepresentation of medical science by the authors of the HCHSCRO led to negative news media coverage; by embracing a sensationalist, media-aimed stance, the salient content of the Report was eclipsed by its own 'attention-grabbing' headlines. *The Daily Mirror*'s headline of June 10th summed up the episode as 'a big fat lie' (Gilfeather, 2004). Thus the HCHSCRO (2004) had been publically discredited. The media attention that the Report had stimulated did not influence the obesity policy agenda, and might even have reduced public trust in governmental responses to population obesity. The Report had, however, contributed to the development of proposals for action on obesity set out in the White Paper 'Choosing Health – Making Healthy Choices Easier' (2004). The White Paper called for a cross-governmental approach, but couched obesity prevention and reversal in terms of a series of lifestyle choices for individuals and communities.

Foresight: Tackling Obesities – Future Choices 2007

Like the House of Commons Health Select Committee Report on Obesity, 2004, the Foresight Report 'Tackling Obesities: Future Choices' (Butland et al., 2007) was concerned with the health costs of rising obesity rates. This time, however, the costs were projected into the future, to 2050, and obesity was conceived of as a complex problem (Finegood et al., 2010). The aim of the Foresight (2007) project was to examine how the UK could respond sustainably to the increasing prevalence of obesity by the year 2050. A systems mapping approach was used to gain insight into the biological and social complexity of obesity, and an obesity system map was constructed using detailed advice from a large group of experts drawn from several different disciplines. According to the map's authors and constructors (Butland et al., 2007; Chipperfield et al., 2007), it represented the most comprehensive 'whole systems' view of the determinants of energy balance. In the foreword to the document, Sir David King, then Chief Scientific Adviser to the British Government and Head of the Government Office for Science, stated that:

> Extensive media coverage has ensured that we're all aware that obesity is on the increase. But popular views on the issue all too often draw on stereotypes, present simplified descriptions of the problem, and have an unrealistic assessment of the solutions. These oversimplifications do not reflect the current state of scientific evidence and understanding. Nor do they help Government develop and implement a sustained response to a problem that will have profound long-term consequences for health and well-being and major costs to the health budget and the wider economy. (King, 2007: 1)

The document reported on obesity prevalence in the UK and its costs to the economy. It stated that the obesity epidemic could not be prevented by individual action alone and demanded a societal approach involving changes at multiple levels: personal, familial, communal and national. It also stated that tackling obesity required partnerships between government, science, business and civil society. The words of Sir David King in his Foreword place the construction of an obesity system map as central to developing more complex thinking about obesity and its control:

> The work reported here represents an independent scientific enquiry into the complex system of factors contributing to obesity – the system map, included in this report, is the first attempt to capture this complexity schematically. Futures thinking, through scenario planning and the quantitative model developed for Foresight, has allowed the exploration of longer-term trends and demonstrates that achieving change will require patience and persistence. (King, 2007: 1)

Novelty in this report consisted of its presentation of population obesity as being complex and systemic, and less due to individual responsibility. Despite this, most of the media coverage focused on the rising rates of obesity in the UK and their economic costs. The BBC reported that the economic cost of obesity had been significantly over-estimated by the Foresight team, and questioned the basis upon which obesity was calculated (Vadon, 2007). As previously, journalists emphasized lifestyle factors, nutrition and individual behaviour as being key to explaining the rise in obesity rates in Britain. However, the notion of passive obesity, introduced in the Foresight Report, was picked up by the *Guardian* and *Observer* newspapers, which reported on market-liberal structures as affecting obesity rates (Campbell, 2007). This was a new way of packaging older discourses about obesity and lifestyle factors, but with a twist: individual responsibility was not to blame, as environmental factors conducive to the development of obesity were extremely strong and difficult to resist. However, individual behaviour continued to be central in articles on the Foresight Report within the health and diet sections of UK newspapers, and the Foresight map was little mentioned, perhaps because it was non-intuitive and difficult to decipher (cf. Goodchild & Lydall, 2007; Martin, 2007; Smith, 2007). The notable exception was an attack on the authors of the Foresight Report and the map for its unintelligibility from the pharmaceutical correspondent for the *Financial Times*, Andrew Jack (2007), in *The Lancet*.

News reporting of the Foresight Report disseminated part of what was novel about the report, and sometime took a critical stance towards scientific and policy authorities, including those that generated the report itself. However, the news media largely ignored what was most difficult, the systems map; where the map did receive coverage, the reporting was critical of the authorities that produced the map. This revealed the tension between the news media's ethos of reporting on what is novel, and the need to make reporting relatable to readers, such that novelty must be reduced to (and sometimes obscured by) familiar rhetoric, commensurate with the public's accepted 'knowledge' and 'common-sense'. The ways in which the news media framed obesity did not change markedly: obesity remained a crisis, but perhaps less subject to individual control than had been previously emphasized. Systemic causes involving multiple actors, although very heavily emphasized in the report, received comparatively little attention. However, with a change in government in mid-2010, a reaffirmation of earlier individualist values was again reflected in policy papers.

Healthy Lives, Healthy People – A Call to Action on Obesity in England (2011)

The white paper 'Healthy lives, healthy people – our strategy for public health in England' was published in November 2010, after a hurried period of consultation and advisory meetings initiated by the Conservative-Liberal Democrat coalition. This document was aimed at increasing public involvement in health initiatives in the UK, across all areas of concern, and across the lifespan. Obesity was an integral part of this, as an important predisposing risk factor for a range of chronic diseases. In mid-October 2011, the Department of Health released an affiliate report, 'Healthy lives, healthy people – a call to action of obesity in England' (2011). The report challenged businesses to help play a greater role, alongside government and non-governmental organizations, to change environments so that individuals could make healthier choices, which could then contribute to reductions in excessive body weight. It also called on the food and drink industry to extend and intensify efforts to help people make healthier choices, to empower local communities in making public health decisions, and to reduce the dietary energy intakes of the national population.

At the same press conference, on the same day, the Scientific Advisory Committee on Nutrition also launched a report. This was a technical report on the dietary energy requirements of the British population, which was unproblematic in itself, but which led to muddled reporting by journalists when considered in combination with the 'Call to Action on Obesity' report. Most articles reported on the continued rise in UK obesity rates, and its current and future economic costs. Some found 'Healthy Lives, Healthy People' to be nonsensical and engaging in avoidance, and even chose to ridicule it. For example, the *London Evening Standard*'s front page headline for that day, in response to the October 13th launch, was: 'Obesity crisis solved: Eat less' (Cecil & Randhawa, 2011). *The Guardian* newspaper recruited celebrity chef Jamie Oliver to trash the report, calling the strategy 'worthless, regurgitated, patronising rubbish' and saying that '[s]imply telling people what they already know – that they need to eat less and move more – is a complete cop-out' (Boseley, 2011). The media also criticized Health secretary Andrew Lansley's statement at the press conference that he would seek a responsibility deal with the food and beverage industries that would involve them making voluntary reductions in the energy density of their products.

The media launch of this Report was misinterpreted, but had again drawn attention to a different approach to obesity, this time seeking partnership with food corporations. The Responsibility Deal Food Network was subsequently formed by a number of major food corporations operating in the UK, including Coca-Cola, the Kellogg Company, Danone, Sainsbury, Kraft Foods, Nestlé, Tate & Lyle, Unilever and Pepsico, to work towards a joint energy-density reduction goal for their products.

Obesity and Reporting Governmental Obesity Documents

Since 2001, obesity rates have carried on increasing in most age and gender groups in the UK, although at slower rates than in the previous two decades (Wang et al., 2011). It is impossible to tell how much impact, if any, government policy on obesity control has had on these patterns. Public health policies towards halting or slowing down the rising prevalence of obesity seem ineffective (Lake and Townsend, 2006), and recent times have seen the growth of demands for radical and holistic but sustained efforts that go beyond public health to reverse this trend (Omoleke, 2011). The failure of current public health interventions may be due to inconsistent, non-sustained, fragmented anti-obesity measures, poor understanding of the ecology of obesity (until recently), the societal normalization of obesity, and a lack of strong political will to convert research findings into actions, especially if such actions might impact on economic interests (Omoleke, 2011). British governments of lesser and greater market-liberal economic persuasion have struggled with controlling obesity rates, and seem to have failed. Perhaps this is because market-liberalism itself contributes to the obesity epidemic (Offer et al., 2010). Interestingly, there is largely an absence of news media critiques of such policy failure, although the recent policy movement toward fostering social responsibility among food corporations, to reduce the energy density of foods, has been met with media criticism.

Governmental reports on obesity and obesity policy are important, at least to take stock and reappraise what appears to be a failing campaign. For the news media, the release of such reports provides an opportunity to refresh or re-run their positions on the issue. The four case studies given show that obesity reporting by the news media has a set of parameters (for example, rising rates, economic costs, personal responsibility, environmental factors) that varies a little according to the political leanings and intended audience of the publication. When a governmental report aims to be quite radical, as with the Foresight Report (2007), in its engagement with complexity, journalistic reporting simplifies or entirely avoids it. When trying to use the news media device of sensationalism, as in the House of Commons Health Select Committee Report on Obesity (2004), errors were quickly identified and the government attacked or ridiculed. Criticism or ridicule may be the price to be paid by government for attempting to keep the policy agenda on obesity at the forefront of public consciousness, while trying to shape the framing of obesity by the news media.

Government reports on obesity are released to the news media with various aims, including: 1) highlighting the importance of the problem, with a call to arms to address it; 2) emphasizing where responsibility lies for fixing the problem (often not placed with government but with other agencies); and 3) creating the right public opinion for change. The release of the four reports described in this article addressed, largely successfully, the first two of these aims, but in varying and (in the case of the House of Commons Health Select Committee Report on Obesity 2004*)* unexpected ways. Given the high and rising obesity rates in the UK, the issue clearly affects the public, but the complexity of population obesity makes it difficult for journalists to bring agencies and institutions to task over it. At the time of writing, however, the drive towards the responsible marketing of foods to prevent childhood obesity has brought major food corporations under greater media scrutiny. It is perhaps a politically nifty trick to try to shift media presentations of responsibility for obesity away from government (obesity as a health and economic problem) and the individual (obesity as a lifestyle and health issue) to the corporations themselves (obesity as an outcome of market-liberal forces and corporate social irresponsibility). Yet making food corporations responsible for ethical marketing practices might prove to be as unwise as putting the banks in charge of their own regulation.

References

Association for the Study of Obesity (2011). *Obesity policy in England.* Kent: Deal.

Bonfiglioli, C., Smith, B.J., King, L., et al. (2011). Risky exercise – is physical activity losing the news race? *Australian Journalism Review, 33(1)*, 73–84.

Boseley, S. (2011, October 13). Jamie Oliver brands Andrew Lansley obesity plan 'patronising rubbish'. *The Guardian.* Retrieved from http://www.theguardian.com/society/2011/oct/13/uk-five-billion-calories-obesity.

Butland, B., Jebb, S., Kopelman, P., et al. (2007). *Foresight. Tackling obesities: Future choices project report.* London: Government Office for science.

Campbell, D. (2007, October 14). Obesity crisis to cost £45bn a year. *The Observer.* Retrieved from http://www.theguardian.com/society/2007/oct/14/health.medicineandhealth.

Cecil, N. & Randhawa, K. (2011, October 13). Obesity crisis solved: Eat less, says Health Secretary. *London Evening Standard.* Retrieved from http://www.standard.co.uk/news/obesity-crisis-solved-eat-less-says-health-secretary-6453337.html.

Chipperfield, T., O'Brien, R., Bolderson, T., et al. (2007). Visualising the future: Scenarios to 2050. Foresight Tackling Obesities: Future Choices. Retrieved from http://www.foresight.gov.uk.

Entman, R.M. (1993) Framing: Toward clarification of a fractured paradigm. *Journal of Communications, 43*, 51–58.

Finegood, D.T., Merth, D.T.N. & Rutter, H. (2010). Implications of the foresight obesity system map for solutions to childhood obesity. *Obesity, 18*, S13–S16.

Gilfeather, P. (2004, June 10). A big fat lie: 'Obese' girl had genetic disorder. *Daily Mirror.*

Goodchild, S. & Lydall, R. (2007, October 17). London 2012 will be 'unhealthy games'. *London Evening Standard.* Retrieved from http://www.standard.co.uk/news/london-2012-will-be-unhealthy-games-6638802.html.

Jack, A. (2007). Obesity plan lacks foresight. *The Lancet, 370*, 1528–1529.

King, D. (2007). Foreword. In B. Butland, S. Jebb, P. Kopelman, et al., *Foresight. Tackling obesities: Future choices project report.* London: Government Office for science.

Lake, A. & Townshend, T. (2006). Obesogenic environments: Exploring the built and food environments. *Journal of The Royal Society for the Promotion of Health, 126*, 262–267.

Lang, T. & Rayner, G. (2007). Overcoming policy cacophony on obesity: An ecological public health framework for policymakers. *Obesity Reviews, 8 (supplement 1)*, 165–181.

McCombs, M. & Shaw, D. (1972). The agenda-setting function of mass media. *Public Opinion Quarterly, 36*, 176–87.

Martin, D. (2007, October 17). Obesity: Deadlier than smoking; Being fat can knock 13 years off your life. *Daily Mail.*

Meikle, J. (2001, February 15). Action urged to cut the fat of the land: Poor diet and lack of exercise blamed for rise in obesity. *The Guardian.* Retrieved from http://www.theguardian.com/society/2001/feb/15/publichealth.uknews.

Musingarimi, P. (2008). *Obesity in the UK: A review and comparative analysis of policies within the devolved regions.* London: International Longevity Centre.

Northrop, M. (n.d.). *The social amplification of risk in relation to obesity.* University of Kent: Social Context and Responses to Risk.

Offer, A., Pechey, R. & Ulijaszek, S. (2010). Obesity under affluence varies by welfare regimes: The effect of fast food, insecurity, and inequality. *Economics & Human Biology, 8(3)*, 297–308.

Omoleke, S. (2011). Obesity: A major public health challenge of 21st century in the United Kingdom (UK). *Journal of Public Health and Epidemiology, 3*, 560–566.

Picard, R.G. & Yeo, M. (2011). *Medical and health news and information in the UK media: The current state of knowledge.* Oxford: Reuters Institute for the Study of Journalism.

Sanders, T. (2004). Select committee castigated for citing death of 3 year old girl in obesity report. *British Medical Journal, 328*, 1503.

Smith, R. (2007, October 17). Half of adults 'will be obese by 2050'. *The Telegraph.* Retrieved from http://www.telegraph.co.uk/news/uknews/1566436/Half-of-adults-will-be-obese-by-2050.html.

Vadon, R. (2007, November 22). Cost of obesity 'over-estimated'. *BBC News: Radio 4's The Investigation.* Retrieved from http://news.bbc.co.uk/1/hi/health/7106219.stm.

Wang, Y.C., McPherson, K., Marsh, T., et al. (2011). Health and economic burden of the projected obesity trends in the USA and the UK. *The Lancet, 378(9793)*, 815–825.

Wheldon, J. (2004, May 27). Child, 3, dies from being too fat. *Daily Express*.

Chapter 10

Heavy Viewing: Emergent Frames in Contemporary News Coverage of Obesity[1]

Helene A. Shugart

In the last decade, obesity has come to occupy a central role in the public imagination and on the national agenda. Why this is so is likely attributable to a host of reasons: Schwarz (1986) has noted that, historically and today, national public interest in obesity is allegorical, increasing commensurate with concerns about material abundance and (over)consumption eroding the country's moral integrity. Similarly, Levy-Navarro (2008) argues that contemporary concerns about obesity may be fuelled by broader concerns regarding national strength and fitness – figurative and literal – in a context of international threat and instability. Still others (e.g., Nestle, 2002; Finkelstein & Zuckerman, 2008) suggest that industry is heavily implicated in promoting obesity in the interest of profit, from flooding the food market with cheap, calorie-dense, and nutritionally empty foods to responding to novel material needs of an increasingly obese population in the form of drugs, assistance programmes, and furniture. Certainly, the high health and economic tolls incurred by obesity (e.g., Finkelstein & Zuckerman; Gard & Wright, 2005; 'Health, United States', 2006; 'Obesity and Overweight', 2008) have prompted the US Surgeon General to characterize obesity as an 'epidemic' and, more ominously, as 'the terror within' – not only on a par with but soon to overtake terrorism as the greatest threat to the nation ('Obesity Bigger Threat Than Terrorism?' 2006). Similarly, the CDC asserts that the 'obesity epidemic' poses a greater threat to the US population than weapons of mass destruction (Fox, 2003). These and other health entities have launched a number of public campaigns and initiatives designed to raise awareness and provide redress, primarily in the form of educating the public about proper nutrition and exercise.

Taking their cue from this alarmist tone and ensuing measures, the news media have followed suit in terms of positioning obesity prominently in coverage: Lawrence (2004) noted a fivefold increase in national news coverage of obesity between the years of 1992 and 2003, and Kim and Willis (2007) and Saguy and Almeling (2008) have respectively noted that mainstream news coverage of obesity has increased further since Lawrence completed her study. These critics, among a small handful of others across disciplines, have assessed how obesity has been

1 Reprinted from Shugart, H.A. (2011). Heavy Viewing: Emergent Frames in Contemporary News Coverage of Obesity. *Health Communication*, 26(7), 635–648.

'framed' in news coverage, operating from the established premise that persistent and pervasive frames, or 'organizing principles [regarding an issue] that ... work symbolically to meaningfully structure the social world' (Reese, 2003: 11) in news coverage, can shape audience perception of and even behaviour as relevant to that issue (Entman, 1993; Iyengar, 1991; Scheufele, 1999).

Because the matter of obesity is so salient today, and because framing of the issue may have a considerable effect on public perceptions, practices, and policies, regular, periodic assessment of the framing of obesity in mainstream news coverage is warranted. In that spirit, this study assesses news coverage of obesity in mainstream news outlets aired or published between June 2008 and December 2009. Utilizing qualitative content analysis combined with discourse analysis, I identified and assessed prominent common themes and patterns in the framing of obesity across these texts. Representing a departure from previous findings, this analysis revealed fatalism to be the predominant theme characterizing obesity in recent contemporary mainstream news coverage, signalling an overarching *Zeitgeist* frame that destabilizes the heretofore widely recognized binary of episodic and thematic frames that undergird framing theory and analyses. Accordingly, this study prompts a reconsideration and elaboration of key tenets of framing theory. By extension, the fatalistic theme and *Zeitgeist* frame trouble the environmental/individual attribution binary that has long dominated public discourses around health issues in general, including obesity. These findings may suggest shifting cultural attitudes regarding obesity and perhaps even health more broadly and may hold significant implications for the shaping of public policies, campaigns, and initiatives.

Health Attributes

In 1980, Robert Crawford identified 'healthism' as a form of medicalization and a perspective prevalent in advanced capitalist societies that sites the problem(s) of and solutions to health and disease at the level of the individual. Accordingly, health is a matter of personal responsibility; implicitly, then, it is rendered a moral issue, insofar as disease is articulated as symptomatic of *ir*responsibility. That is, 'the person is the victim of her/his health turned nasty, but also the agency responsible for this state of affairs' (Fox, 1993: 135).

As a number of critics have observed, this perspective is ideologically charged and politically consequential (e.g., Crawford, 1980; Lupton, 1995; Tesh, 1994; Waitzkin, 1991). That is, locating health exclusively or even primarily within the realm of personal responsibility obfuscates myriad social, structural, and institutional factors that contribute to health and illness in powerful and complex ways, ranging from demographic factors such as class, gender, race/ethnicity, and ability to (often interrelated) literal matters of access: for example, to information, resources, and health care. Furthermore, casting health in terms of personal responsibility summarily deflects a consideration of the role of institutions in addressing those social and material considerations. As Zoller (2008) notes, the 'lifestyle theory of causation', which posits health as an outcome of one's everyday behaviours and practices, has considerable cultural traction as an ostensible alternative (to individual) theory of health. However, while it arguably mitigates the conscious agency suggested by the personal responsibility model, it 'operates similarly [to that model] to maintain the status quo by directing attention toward the individual and away from political and social contexts' (392).

In contrast to the individualization and privitization of health asserted by that model, environmental theories that emphasize the ecological dimensions (an admittedly broad category, which could variously encompass structural, sociopolitical, and lifestyle aspects) of health and disease have been articulated by scholars across disciplines. Although these theories are gaining some ground (e.g., Barry et al., 2009; Kersh, 2009; Lawrence, 2004), this is relative: they continue to have significantly less resonance in public discourses about health. Furthermore, as Tesh (1994) argues, environmental explanations tend to be taken up in discrete terms, often as relevant exclusively to 'lifestyle', thus slipping readily into a theory of health as an individual matter and, again, eliding more abstract, diffuse, and complex considerations that would call for structural and/or institutional redress. Zoller (2008) notes that currently popular 'multicausal web' or multifactorial health promotion efforts, which ostensibly integrate individual and environmental considerations as relevant to health, realize this slippage and in fact reify the binary insofar as they 'fail to prioritise structural and political issues, making discrete changes and easier choice for decision makers' (393). Finally, while a handful of critics (e.g., Lupton, 1995; Peterson & Lupton, 1996; Tesh, 1994) have advocated for a radical approach to public health that 'prioritises interventions in sociopolitical power' (Zoller, 2008: 393), that perspective has (perhaps obviously) not featured significantly, if at all, in public discourses about health.

Clearly, the binary of individual and environmental explanations for health and disease is pervasive, and individual theories remain markedly more ubiquitous. Even ostensibly environmental theories tend to conflate with the rhetoric of personal responsibility by dint of emphasizing discrete 'choices' and 'lifestyles' as loci for practical action. A primary motivation for this study was to assess whether and how that binary continues to be manifest, specifically as relevant to news coverage of obesity. My findings – that fatalism constitutes the predominant theme in that coverage, parlaying into an overarching *Zeitgeist* frame – suggest a rather novel development in light of the heretofore governing binary. That is, this framing greatly diffuses the narrative of personal responsibility for health and arguably more effectively integrates individual and environmental explanations insofar as it does not eventually reduce down to the discrete level of personal responsibility. As will be demonstrated, this is not necessarily a positive development, however, at least not in the case of the news coverage analysed; nonetheless, this study suggests a marked turn in the public discourse about obesity and possibly about health more broadly. The implications of that turn for public health – both negative and positive – warrant attention.

Mediating Obesity

As obesity has increasingly captured the public imagination, a number of scholars across disciplines have taken up the matter from various perspectives and with various aims. Working from the assumption that obesity is a problem, several scholars question the 'moral panic' engendered by designating obesity as an 'epidemic' or 'crisis', noting that a number of institutions – including private, political, medical, and media – stand to gain considerably from such a designation (Gard & Wright, 2005; Levy-Navarro, 2008; Schwarz, 1986). Representing quite different ends of the disciplinary and political spectrum of obesity research, economists have tracked specifically how rising rates of obesity affect the economy both negatively and positively (e.g., Finkelstein & Zuckermann, 2008), and cultural critics have assessed the ways in which obesity functions politically to mark identity in oppressive ways (e.g., LeBesco, 2004; Sobal & Maurer, 1999). Within the field of health communication, a few scholars have addressed popular mediated representations of obesity, for example as articulated in magazines (Campo & Mastin, 2007), celebrity coverage (Ferris, 2003), and prime-time programming (Kline, 2003; Shugart, 2010; Signiorelli, 1993). Each of these studies takes up, in various ways, how the causes of and/or solutions to obesity are articulated in respective media fare; across these contexts, the studies found that personal responsibility was found to be overwhelmingly articulated, variations relevant to the degree and kind of responsibility attendant to certain conditions (such as race, gender, and/or class) notwithstanding. But marginally more scholarly attention to mediated representations of obesity, both within and outside of the field of health communication, has been directed toward news coverage, more specifically to how obesity is or has been framed in that coverage. In these studies, the matter of individual responsibility is overwhelmingly engaged as a 'frame'.

Broadly speaking, 'frames' refer to the ways in which individuals organize and make sense of their impressions, experiences, and perceptions of the world (Hallahan, 1999; Reese, 2003). Perhaps obviously, compelling frames typically reflect or resonate with an individual's cultural knowledge, for 'frames are embedded in cultural and symbolic systems and communicate values and beliefs that are meaningful in those systems' (Connolly-Ahern & Broadway, 2008: 366). The issue of framing is thus relevant to myriad contexts, but it has been taken up by media scholars as a theoretical and methodological perspective to the end of examining the effects of mediated representations. In this context, critics seek to identify and assess consistent and compelling patterns that characterize the representation(s) of a given issue in media fare. Although framing studies can be conducted as relevant to various media venues, formats, and genres, the bulk of critical attention has been directed to news framing in particular, given its relevance to the agenda setting function of the news and the particular salience attributed to the issue of representing 'reality', as news content typically purports and is perceived to do (Entman, 1993; Scheufele, 2000). Gitlin (1980) avers that news frames constitute 'tacit little theories about what exists, what happens and what matters' (6–7) and thus feature particular significance for the shaping of public understandings and attitudes; more specifically, Entman asserts that 'to frame is to select some aspects of a perceived reality and make them more salient in a communicating text, in such a way as to promote a particular problem definition, causal interpretation, moral evaluation and/or treatment recommendation' (52).

In general, news framing studies have overwhelmingly addressed coverage of political, technological, and scientific issues. Comparatively, news framing analyses of health-related issues have been relatively sparse to date (Shih, Wijaya & Brossard, 2008: 142), an oversight that warrants redress insofar as 'media reflect and interact with the public's understanding of a health issue' (Connolly-Ahern & Broadway, 2008: 367). In light of Entman's (1991) assertion that news frames craft 'commonsense' understandings of issues, assessing how health issues are framed can illuminate public discourses around health issues, including as they shape everyday perceptions, practices, and even policies relevant to them. Most framing analyses that have been conducted regarding news coverage of health matters have examined 'isolated' issues (Shih, Wijaya & Brossard, 2008: 142), such as fetal alcohol syndrome (Connolly-Ahern & Broadway, 2008), fertility (Shaw & Giles, 2009), and ADHD (Schmitz, Filippone & Edelman, 2003). Of late, a handful of critics have begun attending to the framing of health issues that have captured broad public attention on national and global scales, for example as relevant to health epidemics such as SARS and AIDS (e.g., Luther & Zhou, 2005; Wallis & Nerlich, 2005; Wu, 2006). In this vein, a few scholars have begun to address the framing of obesity in increased news coverage of the issue.

Findings regarding the news framing of obesity, reflective of framing studies more broadly, draw heavily on Iyengar's (1991) distinction between thematic and episodic frames. Iyengar avers that, given the relatively simplistic terms in which news stories tend to be constructed, characterizations of issues tend to feature either episodic frames, wherein a given subject is articulated anecdotally as an isolated or decontextualized event; or thematic frames, through which issues are generally portrayed in such a way as to 'emphasise broader trends or social conditions' (3). Unlike episodic framing, 'thematic framing is thought to foster a sense of shared responsibility and prompt collective action' (Iyengar, 1991: 3) by fostering greater public understanding of the scope and scale of the issue, a dynamic corroborated by a number of studies (e.g., Kersh, 2009; Lawrence, 2004; Major, 2009).

Notably, this binary is highly commensurate with the individual/environmental health attribution binary described above, a commensurability that has been realized in coverage of obesity that has been studied to date. Within the schema of episodic and thematic framing, news coverage of obesity tends to manifest in corresponding frames of either individual responsibility (episodic) or societal or environmental responsibility (thematic). A number of scholars (e.g., Guttman & Ressler, 2001; Salmon, 1989; Wallack et al., 1993) have noted that, in general, individual responsibility tends to be overwhelmingly emphasized in news coverage of health issues, and obesity is no exception. Consistent with noted studies of otherwise mediated depictions of obesity, analyses of news framing of obesity to date have revealed a very strong episodic or personal responsibility bias, as relevant to coverage of both causes of and solutions to obesity – that is, 'fatness is framed as the product of unhealthy choices' (Saguy & Almeling, 2008: 57) and/or of lack of self-discipline and – control (also Kersh, 2009; Kim & Willis, 2007; Lawrence, 2004; Major, 2009). Importantly, several of these scholars have also noted that environmental causes, or thematic frames, appeared to be gaining ground over time. However, this was found to be quite relative, as compared to virtually absent consideration in earlier news coverage (e.g., Kim & Willis). Additionally, 'as claims about an unhealthy food and activity environment have increased, the role of personal responsibility for one's health has been strongly articulated in response' (Lawrence, 2004: 69; also Saguy & Almeling, 2008), thus ultimately reinscribing and reinforcing individual responsibility via a sort of 'backlash' dynamic. These studies definitively assert that a personal responsibility theory continues to supersede environmental explanations in mainstream news coverage of obesity; they also secure the binary of episodic and thematic frames as competing bases in the portrayal of health issues.

My intent with this analysis is to add to these findings by assessing more recent mainstream news coverage of obesity. My finding that fatalism is the predominant theme in mainstream contemporary news coverage of obesity represents a signal departure from prior studies that have clearly situated individual or (less commonly) environmental causes and/or solutions to the articulated 'problem'. The theme of fatalism emergent in more recent news coverage, however, elides this binary – or, in the rare instances in which both models are invoked, bifurcation. This is not to say that personal and/or environmental factors are not referenced in this coverage; to the contrary, they continue to be invoked, often explicitly. However, they are framed in ways that cultivate a perception of obesity and the risk(s) thereof as practically unavoidable.

In fact, fatalism is not a novel construct as relevant to perceptions of health and health risk, and increasing literature in recent years has identified its prevalence among, in particular, ethnic and racial minorities and the poor (e.g., Powe & Johnson, 2005; Mechanic, 2002). Shen et al. (2009) note that 'fatalism can be conceptualized as a set of health beliefs that encompasses such dimensions as predetermination, pessimism and attribution of one's health (life events) to luck' and/or fate, destiny, or spiritual agents (598). Notably, neither individual nor environmental factors are necessarily obviated in this definition, even if they are implicitly rendered as dubious. Certainly, the theme of fatalism identified in this analysis suggests a blending of episodic and thematic frames and, more broadly, of individual and environmental theories of health, albeit in ways that render each wanting in explanatory and practical utility. These findings are thus significant insofar as they can contribute to general awareness and understanding of cultural perceptions and practices of obesity; to shaping campaigns, initiatives, and policies designed to address the rising rates of obesity and associated diseases; and to framing theory more broadly, in terms of troubling the episodic and thematic frames binary on which the bulk of framing theory has generally been predicated historically. Furthermore, this study may signal a trend in broader public discourses regarding health issues away from the parallel binary of individual or environmental attributions, as has largely been the case historically.

Method

The methodological assumptions that inform this project reflect a combination of interpretive, critical, and cultural perspectives. This is an interpretive venture to the extent that I am engaged in assessing the 'construction of meanings related to health and medicine' (Zoller & Dutta, 2008: 6), and my methods of choice – qualitative framing and close textual analysis – speak directly to that endeavour. This is also a critical project to the extent that I am compelled by the question of how power relations are articulated in the texts that I have elected to examine – specifically, relations between the individual, society, and government. More specifically, I am intrigued by the question of who (or what) is advantaged by the patterns of representation revealed in this analysis, and who or what is disadvantaged (e.g., Lupton, 1994; Waitzkin, 1991; Zoller & Kline, 2008). And finally, this is a cultural enterprise insofar as I apprehend the mainstream mediated texts I have selected for this project as both a collective index and purveyor of evolving and dynamic cultural understandings about obesity in particular and health more broadly – a widely shared assumption on the part of cultural critics, including those who increasingly number in the ranks of health communication scholars (e.g., Dutta, 2007; Lupton, 1994, 1995). As Lupton (1994) states, a cultural studies approach to assessing 'the ways in which medical practices and institutions are represented in the mass media ... is integral to ... attempting to understand the socio-cultural aspects of medicine and health-related knowledges and practices', not least insofar as certain perspectives are privileged at the expense of others (17).

For this project, I assessed the news coverage of obesity across mainstream – that is, widely disseminated, well recognized, and thus highly available and accessible – news sources, both print and televised. My intention was to cast as wide a net as possible to encompass the most primary and pervasive sources of news that consumers are likely to encounter. To that end, I selected three primary newspapers that are nationally distributed, either by design or by subscription rates, namely *USA Today* (USAT), *The New York Times* (NYT) and *The Washington Post* (WP); two newsmagazines that boast the broadest national circulation for that genre – *Time* and *Newsweek*; and four mainstream network television stations, ABC, CBS, NBC, and CNN – specifically, relevant portions of their 'regular' evening news broadcasts as well as daily morning shows and weekly newsmagazines. Between the months of June 2008 and December 2009, I identified and selected all in-depth (either 'cut away' broadcasts for a duration of at least 3 minutes or 'long' – 500+ words – print articles) news stories that featured 'obesity' as either a headline or primary term, by either viewing/reading the stories when originally broadcast/printed or locating them through website archives and/or databases utilizing the search term 'obesity'. Within the designated time frame and noted parametres relative to focus and depth of attention, I identified a total of 541 news stories: 157 newspaper stories (USAT 92; NYT 42; WP 23); 103 newsmagazine stories (*Time* 61; *Newsweek* 42); and 281 televised news stories (ABC 72; CBS 76; CNN 93; NBC 40).

The identified news stories engaged the issue of obesity across a range of topics, including, for instance, newly discovered linkages to various diseases; escalating rates of obesity; childhood obesity; drugs to treat obesity; and policies for the treatment of obesity. Procedurally, I attended to purported causes of and solutions to the problem of obesity within these stories, whether explicitly or implicitly engaged. This is salient in terms of tracking whether and, if so, how frames are shifting between thematic and episodic frames – or environmental versus individual explanation for both causes and solutions. At this point, I was engaged in qualitative framing analysis. Qualitative framing analysis, as Connolly-Ahern & Broadway (2008) note, involves repeated and extensive engagement with a text[s] and looks holistically at the material to identify frames' (p. 369). This entailed identifying, via close textual analysis, the 'discourse' of obesity as articulated in the identified texts, or the representations, themes, and patterns of how the causes of and solutions to obesity were framed or portrayed across the selected texts (e.g., Connolly-Ahern & Broadway, 2008; Cooper & Pease, 2009; Shaw & Giles, 2009). Close textual analysis is a natural complement for framing analysis because 'there is an inextricable link between discourses and frames' (Johnston, 1995: 219) insofar as 'frames are themselves discursive strategies designed to construct meaning and "reality"' (McInerny, 2006: 656). Upon careful and repeated viewing and reading of the selected texts, a number of frames became apparent – including nostalgia, cultural identity, and, yes, personal responsibility and environmental factors – but fatalism quickly emerged as the most prominent and pervasive theme across the texts, suggesting a novel and significant development in the framing of obesity in mainstream news coverage and, concomitantly, broader cultural understandings of obesity.

Resigned to Fat(e)

The overarching frame that emerged in this analysis was fatalism, or the notion that the US's already high and escalating rates of obesity are inevitable due to circumstances beyond our reasonable control, whether those circumstances are individual or environmental – or both – in nature. Collectively, 323, or 59.7 per cent, of the 541 print and televised news stories analysed evinced this frame, which was strongly and consistently featured across three primary 'culprits': the contemporary world, genetics, and (ineffective) regulation.

Contemporary Life

A significant number of news stories – 116, or 21.4 per cent – identified the contemporary world as the underlying cause of obesity, both in terms of how the US population has arrived at its current state and why, despite increasing attention to the issue and apparent awareness regarding how to resolve it, the 'obesity epidemic' continues to grow. The basic premise of this coverage, across mainstream print and television sources, is that the shape, demands, and consequences of our everyday lives make it virtually impossible to manage weight. Notably, both individual and environmental explanations for and solutions to obesity are invoked in this coverage, but in such a way that redress is presented as impractical. The specific pitfalls of the contemporary world as relevant to obesity, as identified in these news stories, are technology and labour.

News stories that identify contemporary lifestyles as explanatory of obesity levels in the US tend overwhelmingly to focus on the issue of childhood obesity, and this is especially true as relevant to technology. A handful of stories cite the rise of technologies, at work and at home, as fostering a more sedentary population more broadly, such that 'labour intensive jobs' are being phased out 'in favour of technology', ranging from heavy machinery to computers (Carmichael, 2008b, para. 7; also Bakalar, 2008; Rochman, 2009; Stengel, 2008). Furthermore, this may not be simply a matter of bodies at rest; some stories also identify the 'biological impact of mental work' engendered by the rise of technologies, insofar as stress levels, which are associated with computer tasks, may contribute to obesity (e.g., Bakalar, 2008, para. 5; Kantrowitz & Wingert, 2008). However, the vast majority of such stories specifically identify the deleterious effects of media on children's weight. 'Media bombardment' in general is reported as correlated with higher levels of childhood obesity in that the more hours children spend consuming media of any stripe, the more likely they are to be obese (St George, 2008; also Cruz, 2008). Television and the internet are consistently identified as most culpable: 'the transformation of American homes into high-def, Web-enabled, TiVo-equipped entertainment centres means that children who come home after a largely sedentary day at a school desk spend an average of three more sedentary hours in front of some kind of screen' (Kluger, 2008, para. 9; also Szabo, 2008). Furthermore, content as well as quantity of media fare is liable as regards childhood obesity; significant exposure to fast-food advertisements is perhaps obviously reported as directly correlated with childhood obesity ('Food Ads', 2009; Rabin, 2008b), but modelling the behaviours of popular characters who are sedentary and/or consume unhealthy foods and beverages is similarly reported as implicated (e.g., 'Eye Catching Ads', 2009; Szabo, 2008). While these scenarios certainly suggest an avenue for individual action – i.e., parents could eliminate television and/or computer time for children – coverage often cites the absence of working parents or the configuration of school days, for example the heavy reliance on technologies in the classroom (Cruz, 2008) and the elimination of physical education curriculum (Kluger, 2008). Accordingly, different 'lifestyle' choices and actions are presented as limited in their effectiveness, if not futile, to the extent that they collide with structural and institutional factors. Addressing either dimension, per this coverage, is not sufficient, and addressing both is not possible.

Indeed, at least as significant as the attribution, to a greater or lesser degree, of obesity to technology is the articulation of technology's pervasiveness and inevitability in contemporary life. That is, the efficiency and necessity of school and work technologies that result in greater sedentariness are not challenged in these depictions. While content may be subjected to regulation, itself a highly controversial issue, technology is understood as a – actually, *the* – hallmark of social progress and evolution, such that addressing the problem is relevant to 'limiting' rather than eliminating the use of technology to a reasonable amount of time, a task made enormously difficult insofar as work and school are often shaped by technologies and social/familial networks are increasingly created and maintained via technologies (e.g., Kluger, 2008; Rochman, 2009). Again, individual action is articulated as possible but hampered if not negated by structural factors.

The second prominent way in which obesity is attributed to contemporary lifestyles is as relevant to the demands of work. Much of this is a matter of time, or lack thereof: increased work hours over the last few decades must be balanced with familial obligations, such that people don't have the time to exercise or prepare healthy meals. 'Eating healthily can be expensive and time-consuming – two qualities Americans currently have little appetite for. Hitting up the drive-through is cheap, no-hassle and easy to rationalize' (Summers, 2009, para. 6). Reported exhortations on the part of experts to 'make time to exercise as a family' or to 'take the time to cook with your kids' are imparted directly alongside acknowledgement of the 'time squeeze' experienced by the majority of the US population today (Oliwenstein, 2008, para. 4; also Hellmich, 2009; Losh, 2008). Thus, ostensible individual solutions to health are simultaneously negated by the practical impossibilities presented by structural demands. Again, personal responsibility and environmental theories of obesity are presented as co-implicated, yet in a way that places them in opposition to one another and ultimately imparts a sense of futility regarding the issue.

Relatedly, a number of news stories across venues consistently reported findings that obesity is linked to stress, and more specifically cortisol ('stress hormone') levels, implicitly and often explicitly connected to the demands of balancing work and life. In a sort of double whammy, 'longer commutes and more time spent at work and on the computer have made for more sedentary lives [and lead to] greater levels of stress and depression', all factors that are strongly correlated with rising rates of obesity (Rabin, 2009a, D:5). In particular, stress is lined to 'visceral fat', which is 'dangerous, and difficult to lose. It's caused by a lot of things, including cortisol, a hormone produced when we're under stress. You can cut calories and exercise religiously, and still have visceral belly fat, and lots of it' ('Start Saying Goodbye', 2008). Furthermore, this is a vicious cycle: cortisol is suspected of promoting fat, and fat cells in turn generate higher levels of cortisol (Raymond, 2009; Walsh, 2008). The attendant advice – that 'working stress-reduction techniques into your busy days can really help' (Grumman, 2009, para. 12) – clearly acknowledges that stress is likely a consequence of struggling to balance work/life demands, which are just as clearly articulated as inevitable – the above quote assumes as given 'busy days'. In a similar vein, a very prominent news story during the time period surveyed was the finding that obesity is strongly correlated to lack of sufficient sleep, which is frequently attributed to busy lifestyles: 'disturbed sleep or lack of sleep, which many of us regularly experience, leads to disregulation of eating' (Brownell, 2009; also Bakalar, 2009; 'Irregular Sleeping', 2009). Here, too, the common experience of insufficient rest is implicitly articulated as a fact of life today.

As with coverage of the relationship between obesity and technology, what is notable about this coverage is the characterization of work/life balance difficulties as essentially inevitable, simply the nature of the beast that is our contemporary world. While coverage in this vein does not obviate and in fact sometimes explicitly recommends 'making life changes', such as scaling back work hours, relocating, and/or changing professions to the end of avoiding technology, lengthy commutes, and alleviating attendant stressors while increasing time devoted to healthy meal preparation, activity, and sleep, what is important is that these options are not presented as practical or even realistic in current mainstream news coverage of obesity. Coverage in this vein thus articulates both personal responsibility and environmental theories of obesity, but in a way that positions them against each other. Both are articulated as materially 'real', salient, and relevant; however, discrete individual 'choices' and 'changes', the only options proffered, are effectively negated in the face of the demands and constraints of contemporary life, which are in turn articulated as immutable. They are framed in relation to each other in ways that convey hopelessness rather than possibility.

Biological Determinants

Another avenue through which fatalism is realized in contemporary news reports on obesity is via coverage of biological factors, which comprised 112, or 20.7 per cent, of the 541 news stories assessed. Much of this coverage was devoted to reporting the existence of the 'obesity gene' that some individuals possess, which makes them very likely to gain weight and very unlikely to lose it: individuals with a 'common variation of the gene tend to overeat high-calorie foods' ('Study', 2008, para. 1). The inevitability of this relationship, as well as the futility of fighting it, is established by the notion that DNA 'programmes' an individual (Gupta, 2008a), and it is further underscored by articulation of the fact that the obesity gene, also anointed the 'thrifty gene', is an evolutionary product, 'a protection in times of famines past but a risk factor in an [environment] of caloric abundance' (Walsh, 2008, para. 1). Although some coverage in this vein reports that biology is not destiny and that exercise and diet can offset genetic tendencies, suggesting the efficacy of personal responsibility, such recommendations are significantly qualified by the daunting degree of effort and vigilance described as required and even acknowledged as impractical for most people: for the 'time deprived', the 'more intense work needed to improve fitness and lose weight' is less realistic or feasible than the 'modest amount of exercise that can deliver general health benefits' (Schneider, 2008, HE03). This impracticality is captured and underscored by reports that traditional Amish individuals, who evidently possess the 'fat gene', manage to stay trim due to their 'rural nineteenth century lifestyle', which entails 3–4 hours of vigorous activity a day (Heisley, 2008, para. 3; also Park, 2008), a lifestyle that is far removed indeed from the average consumer of such reporting. Furthermore, a number of reports note that even such herculean efforts are ineffective in the long term: a 'draconian diet' characterized by denial of certain foods or calorie restriction almost always results in regaining lost weight (Carmichael, 2008a), and

> pushing people to exercise more [could] actually be contributing to our obesity problem … [b]ecause exercise depletes not just the body's muscles but the brain's self-control "muscle" as well, [leading] many of us [to] feel greater entitlement to eat a bag of chips during that lazy time after we get back from the gym. This explains why exercise could make you heavier … It's likely that I am more sedentary during my nonexercise hours than I would be if I didn't exercise with such Puritan fury. (Cloud, 2009, para. 28)

The crux of this coverage is that fat is biologically preordained in many if not most people, and nothing less than herculean effort – requiring drastic changes if not a full opting out of contemporary life – can alter that. A variation of this theme is apparent in coverage that reports that it is possible to be 'fat but fit', or 'metabolically healthy'. That is, 'despite their excess pounds, many overweight and obese adults have healthy levels of "good" cholesterol, blood pressure, blood glucose and other risks for heart disease' (Parker-Pope, 2008, para. 3). While this finding may or may not be accurate, its characterization in news coverage implicitly underscores the inevitability of fat – 'there's just no fighting the natural rhythms or shapes of one's body' (Kingsbury, 2008, para. 5). Such coverage furthermore suggests that the right kind of fat (subcutaneous or 'brown' fat) – of the sort that our ancestors may have gained via a more 'whole foods' diet – is not only not harmful but may be beneficial (e.g., Springen, 2008). Again, while these reported findings may well be accurate, and they arguably signal a progressive departure from the stigma historically associated with obesity in mediated representations, they reinforce a fatalistic frame by reinscribing the reported evolutionary tendency to gain weight. While individual actions to 'fight obesity' are not obviated in such coverage and are even explicitly endorsed in some cases, they are framed in ways that suggest a futile battle – in this case, against the formidable forces of nature.

Among the news stories that addressed the genetic angle of obesity, a significant number centred upon women in particular, in two notable ways. First, in keeping with the evolutionary frame noted above, women are reported as less able to control their appetites – they are genetically programmed to gain weight more readily and hang on to it longer than men in order to ensure fertility, successful pregnancy, and breastfeeding of infants. That is, 'lower' body fat or a 'pear shape', which is more prevalent in women, is genetically programmed due to its beneficial nature: 'once you store that fat, you don't get rid of it, it pretty much stays there except for extreme circumstance, maybe, maybe starvation let's say, or breast feeding. On the other hand, it also seems to produce inflammation factors, factors that actually block the inflammation and then lower the risk of heart disease and diabetes' ('How Fat Can Be Healthy', 2009; also Rabin, 2009b). Again, this coverage underscores the predestination of weight gain, among women at least. Another way in which women feature in coverage of genetic links to obesity is apparent in reports that what and how much pregnant women eat may 'programme' their children to gain weight in particular ways, in that 'an overweight pregnant woman [may] be creating an environment inside her uterus that predisposes her child to put on fat more quickly than the offspring of normal-weight mothers' (Wingert & Kantrowitz, 2009, para. 3; also Begley, 2009). This secures the notion that individuals (as opposed to their mothers) are not responsible for their weight issues but also obfuscates the significance of environmental factors by suggesting that the die are cast well before one's birth; as one news article asserts, 'If these theories are confirmed, we may come to view pregnancy not as a nine-month wait for the big event but as the crucible of a major health problem, obesity's ground zero' (Paul, 2008). The bottom line in this coverage is, again, that one's obesity is biologically preordained, and subsequent lifestyle changes are implicitly or explicitly described as ineffectual:

> Perhaps an "obese" environment in the womb alters the wiring of the developing brain so as to interfere with normal appetite control, fat deposition, taste in food, or metabolism. Studies on other animals suggest that parts of the brain that control appetite develop differently under "obese" conditions. And in humans, one study has found that babies born to obese mothers have lower resting metabolic rates than babies whose mothers are of normal weight … If this is right, it raises the alarming possibility that the obesity epidemic has a built-in snowball effect. If children born to obese mothers are … predisposed to obesity, they may find staying thin especially hard. (Judson, 2008, WK10)

On the other hand, pregnant women *are* implicitly articulated as culpable, a contemporary manifestation of historical positioning of mothers as the 'moral guardians' of children's health (Lupton, 1995: 42). Notably, however, they are rarely explicitly charged in this coverage; indeed, they typically reflect a vague, abstract, passive persona (as opposed to person*age*). For instance, references are frequently made to 'maternal weight' and 'maternal obesity' rather than particular women (e.g., Park, 2009a; also Paul, 2008), and when particular women are invoked, personal responsibility is offset by noting that, for instance, 'these women may be suffering from undiagnosed diabetes' (Park, 2009a). In this way, they are arguably conflated with nature, simply a fact of life – also not a novel characterization of motherhood (or women in general), and in this case, again, it works to remove even obvious individual choices and changes from the equation of obesity. Mothers' personal responsibility is arguably further offset – in similar, i.e. 'natural forces' ways – by the widely accepted and oft-reported 'fact', in tandem with some of this coverage, that pregnant women are biologically driven to crave certain foods (e.g., 'Curb Those Cravings', 2009). While one can indeed 'curb cravings', the very point of such coverage is that, again, to do so is to defy nature and biology – a daunting, not to mention by definition unnatural, endeavour.

Finally, considerable coverage of the relationship between food and pleasure functions to secure the inevitability of weight gain among some individuals, at least. That is, several stories reported findings that individuals who are overweight or obese are less likely receive pleasure signals in their brains when they eat (e.g., Kliff, 2008; Layton, 2009; 'Obese Enjoy', 2008). Because humans are genetically programmed to experience pleasure – gratification or satisfaction, minimally – upon eating in order to prompt us to eat, those unable to do so readily are physically compelled to consume more and more, which results in weight gain and obesity: 'The more an individual overeats, the less potent the rewards from eating become and that creates a pattern of overeating' (Kliff, 2008, para. 4). That this condition is reported as a 'genetic disposition' that differs only in degree rather than kind from 'normal' responses to eating suggests the inevitability of this cycle. In a similar vein, some news coverage reported findings that obesity may be due, in part, to varying levels and kinds of microbes in one's digestive tract, microbiota that '[help] regulate the calories the body obtains from food and stores as fat' (Park, 2009b, para. 2; also Stein, 2009). Whether and to what extent gut flora levels are genetically or environmentally (for example, by the types of food one consumes or via use of antibiotics) determined remains unclear, these stories report, imbuing obesity further with a fatalistic frame, at least by dint of the ambiguity that surrounds the finding and certainly in tandem with other coverage that describes obstacles to preventing or overcoming obesity. There is no clear recourse available to the individual in terms of making lifestyle changes, nor is clear environmental redress implicated. Of course, potential drug therapies designed to 'correct' dopamine response or gut microbe levels are implicated by such coverage; by the same token, pending further research, policies regulating certain foods or medical prescriptions could theoretically be enacted. But this does not negate the shared fundamental assertion that obesity is not only a natural but logical consequence of human biology in conjunction with caloric abundance, for at least some if not most of the population.

As with characterizations of contemporary lifestyles, what is notable in the case of news stories that report genetic links to obesity is that neither individual nor environmental causes are advanced as definitively responsible for either bringing about or resolving the issue. Both are implicated to some extent, but neither is articulated as concretely culpable or effective, respectively: theoretically, the individual is capable of resisting or avoiding her/his genetic destiny, but options are reported either as requiring monumental, even impossible effort or as unnatural, or both. Likewise, environmental changes along the lines of ensuring the exclusive presence of whole foods and/or to ensure regulation of the quantity of foods that people consume, is theoretically possible – but practically, legally, or ethically unfeasible. Obesity may well be our biological destiny, these stories suggest, and there isn't much we can do about it, on any front.

Ineffective/Detrimental Regulation

A final way in which the frame of fatalism is conveyed is relevant to regulatory efforts – specifically, their ineffective and/or deleterious effects. News stories in this vein, which constituted 17.6 per cent of coverage, engaged the issue across three contexts: changes to food provision in schools, such as limiting or eliminating 'bad' foods or serving more fruits and vegetables at school lunches (Fortin, 2009; Horowitz, 2008); legislation requiring restaurants to post nutritional information for the foods they serve (Barron, 2008; 'Restaurants', 2008); and altering access to certain foods for low-income neighbourhoods, for instance by banning the establishment of additional fast-food restaurants or by establishing 'green carts', or mobile produce vendors, throughout those neighbourhoods ('L.A. Council', 2008; Mindlin, 2008; Rivera, 2008).

Because policy or regulatory changes generally follow environmental explanations for either or both the cause of and solution to obesity, and because environmental considerations are typically understood as the alternative to individual explanations, it would seem logical that regulatory steps would have been articulated as ineffective because they did not address individual choices and behaviours, accordingly identified as the 'real' problem. However, this was not the case in coverage during the time period analysed. Rather, the matter was deflected in favour of either the regulatory practices' speculative nature or broader negative economic and political impact; furthermore, as other critics have noted (e.g., Tesh, 1994; Zoller, 2008), individual 'lifestyles' are often conflated with and become the basis of environmental explanations and solutions. Many of the news stories reported objections to the regulations on the basis of the fact that they were either downright ineffective, 'not really solving the problem' (Nagourney, 2008, para. 3) or experimental: that is, positive outcomes had not been proven, and implementing dramatic changes entailed considerable cost, in terms of both time and money. After all, 'since the FDA has required nutrition labels on [packaged] food [15 years ago], obesity has skyrocketed' (Gupta, 2008b). More recent attempts were characterized as 'arbitrary', singling out one possible contributing factor (salt, transfats, calories, colas, fried foods, or fast foods) in a fairly capricious fashion; a '"ridiculous", "insane" and wrong-headed approach to solving the national obesity epidemic' (Hellmich, 2008, para. 2); and constituting 'backward voodoo economics' (Rivera, 2008, para. 15). While individual and other environmental factors were implicitly alluded to in these representations – for example, posting nutritional information implies that individuals are expected to take action in response to aid from institutional entities – it is notable the allusions were consistently vague and diffuse. 'Health officials need to act more broadly' (Nagourney, 2008, para. 7) was about as specific as it got, thus deflecting clear articulations of the cause(s) of or solution(s) to obesity.

Many news stories that addressed the matter of regulatory measures as regards obesity similarly sidestepped designations of cause and resolution by noting the negative impact of such regulation with respect to the market or to cultural politics. In the former case, considerable coverage in this vein noted that businesses were likely to be hurt by regulations that required posting of nutritional information, which could drive away customers ('Restaurants', 2008); 'cannibalize' existing grocers' businesses who would now have to compete with city subsidized 'green carts' (Mindlin, 2008, para. 4); and 'unfairly blame' the restaurant industry and penalize franchise owners from opening businesses (fast food restaurants) in low-income neighbourhoods, historically highly profitable areas for such businesses ('L.A. Council', 2008, para. 12). In a different vein but similarly deflective, coverage focused on the fact that such regulations were indicative of inappropriate cultural politics, smacking of 'paternalism' and condescension as relevant to disadvantaged communities (Rivera, 2008) and/or of 'a new and appalling level' of bias and discrimination against obese individuals (Hellmich, 2008, para. 9; also Cloud, 2008) – implying, again, that obesity also is a matter of personal responsibility, which is furthermore implicitly articulated as confounding policy efforts. In a variation on this theme as relevant to venerated cultural traditions, school policies banning long-held annual bake sales as a measure against obesity were covered in such a way as to point up the ridiculous lengths to which regulatory agencies might go: 'there shall be no cupcakes', writes one reporter (Medina, 2009; also Luu, 2009). Again, notable here is the fact that questions regarding the causes of and solutions to obesity are elided in this coverage; attention to the broader impact of these regulations, while not irrelevant, renders obesity a 'given' – a condition impervious to regulation, both in terms of effectiveness and in terms of more 'serious' negative impact. But it is furthermore notable that the sentiments largely reported in news stories covering regulatory policies reflect distinctly neoliberal sensibilities insofar as apparently progressive, socially oriented sentiments are articulated to the end of advocating or implementing decidedly conservative economic policies – or, as in this case, decrying the implementation of socially oriented policies. As relevant to news coverage of obesity in that spirit, this manifests in ways that obviate overtly blaming the individual but similarly obviate market regulation, relegating the matter to a sort of ambiguous limbo between individual responsibility and environmental causes – an ambiguity that is highly consistent with a fatalistic frame.

Discussion

Analysis of recent mainstream news coverage of obesity reveals that fatalism is the prominent frame that characterizes such coverage today. As this study demonstrates, this frame is significant, featured in nearly 60 per cent of coverage analysed and distributed across three primary loci – contemporary life, biological determinism, and ineffective/detrimental legislation. Although the remaining 40.3 per cent of coverage for the most part mirrored traditional patterns that have been identified in previous studies – that is, episodic (personal responsibility) or thematic (environmental causes) frames, with far greater representation of episodic frames – a fatalistic frame appears to have superseded them and in fact appears to be gaining ground. For example, the finding that one's social network is a powerful determinant of one's weight was being widely reported at the time that this study concluded: that is, if at least one friend is obese, irrespective of geographical distance (significant given the increasing relevance of technology assisted social networks), one's risk of becoming obese nearly triples due to evolutionary impulses toward 'behavioral imitation – you copy what people close to you are doing – and shared expectations called "norms"' (e.g., Landau, 2009, para. 8). This news story and the way it is being articulated mirrors the fatalistic frame identified in this analysis insofar as it sidesteps clear attribution to either individual and environmental causes without denying either; that is, one could theoretically make conscious choices regarding whom to befriend, but if one already has an obese friend(s), forms alliances with work colleagues or neighbours by dint of proximity or necessity, or learns after forming a friendship that an 'online' friend is obese, those choices become more complicated and less practical. Such coverage further 'confirms' that obesity is insidious and inevitable.

The identification of this frame is significant for several reasons. In the first place, it represents a departure from the binary frame typologies of individual or environmental causes and/or solutions that have historically characterized news coverage of obesity – and indeed, public discourses (mediated and otherwise) about health more broadly in the US. The fatalistic framing of obesity identified in this study elides pat attributions to either the individual or the environment. This is not to say that either explanation is obviated; on the contrary, they are both implicated and often even explicitly invoked, but in ways that point up the futility of taking either tack. Indeed, they are often positioned as oppositional to each other, insofar as, for instance, individual agency is encouraged and simultaneously articulated as stymied by the structural and institutional realities of everyday life. Likewise, policy changes addressing environmental factors are represented as fruitless to the extent that unreliable individual behaviour is implicated as a contingent factor in said policies' success. And of course, biological and evolutionary explanations go one better, fundamentally articulating the plight against obesity as unnatural, a characterization that is underscored rather than countered by exhortations to herculean efforts on the exercise and diet fronts. What renders this coverage fatalistic, again, is not that individual and environmental theories are dismissed, but rather that they *are* invoked, often explicitly, albeit framed in ways that establish the futility of each, especially by dint of their relation to each other.

A fatalistic frame thus may appear to be progressive to the extent that it melds individual and environmental theories of health, which have historically been neatly (and problematically) bifurcated. Moreover, this fusion arguably tempers historically favoured attributions of personal responsibility for health, which has led to significant stigmatization of illness and disease – certainly the case as relevant to obesity and obese individuals (e.g., Ferris, 2003; Levy-Navarro, 2008; Schwarz, 1986). It could be the case that a fatalistic frame signals a more nuanced and sophisticated understanding of the undeniably complicated issue of obesity, and perhaps of health more broadly, especially given that acknowledgement of both individual and environmental explanations does not mirror the conflation of both into 'lifestyle'. That is, as other critics have noted, environmental explanations for health often lapse into conversations and policies regarding relatively more discrete 'lifestyle' factors, which functions practically as a theory of personal responsibility and ultimately belies consideration of broader structural and environmental issues.

However, while a more thoughtful and complex alternative to the binary is very much in order, a fatalistic frame is not that alternative. Fundamentally and by definition, it deflects and dismisses reflection in favour of resignation; obesity is presented not as malleable, complex, and dynamic but fixed and inevitable. This is certainly realized in the strong articulation of fatalism as relevant to regulations and policies designed to redress obesity, which are overwhelmingly characterized as ineffective and/or wrongheaded. In this regard, fatalism may function as something of a 'middle ground', albeit representing limbo or paralysis more than progressiveness. That is, if stigma entailed by a personal responsibility frame is tempered if not elided via a fatalist frame, so too is the role of industry and government by sidestepping an environmental attribution frame. Moreover, this is accomplished precisely by dint of ostensibly merging both attribution typologies, which in fact reinforces rather than dismantles that unproductive binary.

These findings have further implications for framing theory, as well, as relevant to the broader binary benchmark frames of that theory. That is, this study muddles the distinction between episodic and thematic frames, identified by Iyengar (1991), that constitute the prevalent 'master' frames via which issues are presented in news coverage. Just as fatalism simultaneously blurs and minimizes individual and environmental explanations for obesity, episodic and thematic frames are similarly collapsed and superseded by another frame – an epochal *Zeitgeist* frame, one that locates events and issues within broad, sweeping sociohistorical trends. Coverage of those issues thus assumes a 'social commentary' rather than practical and/or political character, wherein intercession of any sort is circumscribed. It may be the case that this frame comes into play as relevant to issues that are culturally contested at that intersection, as many have noted with respect to obesity, even if episodic frames have been overwhelmingly prevalent in coverage heretofore. This may speak to evolving exigencies and audiences around a particular issue at a particular historical moment (see, e.g., Kirkwood & Brown, 1995). Or it may be the case that *Zeitgeist* frames are emergent in contemporary news coverage more broadly, reflective of sensibilities around current cultural tensions and anxieties regarding agency and its limits. More studies addressing the contemporary coverage of a variety of issues are necessary to assess these and other possibilities.

Although the *Zeitgeist* frame as applied to obesity – i.e., manifest as fatalism – is problematic for the reasons I have noted, it is not without promise as a way to understand and engage health issues. Although she takes up the matter of individual and environmental attributions for health issues more broadly in terms of disease prevention policy, Tesh (1994) makes a very useful distinction between alternative models to that binary, which she identifies as inaccurate and unrealistic (83). On the one hand, she notes that a 'multicausal model', which 'demonstrates that a huge number of phenomena go together to produce illness' (58), better reflects the complexity and interdependence of various factors implicated in health, as well as the wrongheadedness and futility of isolating any singular cause. Indeed, this is somewhat reflective of the frame of fatalism, as a manifestation of an overarching *Zeigeist* frame, identified in this study. But just as I discovered, Tesh notes that a multifactorial model may be as problematic and limited as individual or environmental attribution models primarily because it is paralysing: the numerous contributing factors that drive this model 'make any one preventive action appear insignificant [... thus,] in practice, the multicausal model easily becomes a rationale for not taking action. Since everything is connected to everything, we are apparently hopelessly knotted into our own cultural practices, products, and institutions' (62). However, Tesh advances another model in its stead, one that reflects the virtues of a multifactorial model but sidesteps its shortcomings. This 'structural proposal' model, which 'assume[es] that disease originates in the social structure' (77), is risky insofar as it moves up at least one level of abstraction, but ironically, it provides greater traction for health policy insofar as it assumes that 'whatever makes life better in general also makes it healthier. So [for example], the provision of decent housing, good schools, and satisfying jobs would be a prime means of preventing disease' (79). While a structural model 'directs prevention first to the interaction between government and industry', this is not simply a rearticulation of the environmental attribution frame, nor does it obviate the role of the individual; rather, it requires a reimagined relationship among government, citizens, and industry. The significance of citizens' voices is key to the effectiveness of this model, such that obstacles to health experienced by individuals in their everyday lives become the foundation for health policies (79–82).

Especially as informed by the context of a structural model for health policy, my findings feature implications for practices and policies designed to redress the escalating 'obesity epidemic' in the US. That is, public health initiatives and campaigns that are predicated on either individual behaviours or environmental causes may well be missing the mark. If the broader public discourse – which news representations indisputably play a significant role in shaping – is crafting a cultural understanding of obesity as an inevitable byproduct of our everyday lives, decontextualized dictums to 'eat right and exercise' or regulatory measures to enhance the means to do so are neither compelling nor effective. Campaigns and initiatives might instead locate obesity more broadly in the context of everyday lives and engage *both* agency *and* resources in those terms. In this way, the holistic, complex, and practical potential of a *Zeitgeist* frame – which I contend is coopted, inadvertently or not, in contemporary news coverage of obesity that circumscribes agency and intervention – could be recuperated and moved away from an essentially multifactorial model to one that more closely resembles a structural one, as Tesh (1994) describes. That is, the complex social, cultural, historical, economic, and individual conditions that are all implicated in obesity could be acknowledged, and measures proposed to address it could in turn reflect more thoughtful consideration of those conditions. Accordingly, the locus of practices and policies may shift dramatically, quite literally, to sites that synthesize both agency and resources in the context of the everyday and that are clearly founded in individual experiences: as relevant to ensuring workplace gym facilities, for instance; limiting work hours; requiring and subsidizing child care at gyms; subsidizing urban gardens; providing financial incentives for health and fitness, such as reduced insurance premiums or tax deductions; subsidizing whole foods (other than corn and soybeans); requiring gardening, nutrition, and physical education in school curricula; establishing car-free zones in towns and cities. These are but a few examples, and many may seem impractical, even impossible, as measured against normative assumptions and practices. But they do directly engage what is being articulated, in our news coverage and, increasingly, elsewhere (see, e.g., Barry et al., 2009; Shugart, 2010) as both the causes of obesity and the obstacles to its redress – which are not necessarily inaccurate, if they are problematically rendered. Furthermore, they do not facilely indict either individuals or industry but acknowledge the roles of both – indeed, more accurately and importantly, they challenge that binary – in broader social and cultural structures. Rather than bemoan *Zeitgest*, the apparent emergent frame of choice, it could well be taken up and mobilized in ways that acknowledge the infinitely complex, complicated, and convoluted matters of health.

References

Bakalar, N. (2008, September 15). I think, therefore I am fat? *New York Times* [archived web transcript]. Retrieved from http://www.nytimes.com/2008/09/16/health/research/16beha.html?_r=1&scp=88&sq=obesity&st=nyt.

Bakalar, N. (2009, January 1). Children: Study ties too little sleep to too much obesity. *New York Times* [archived web transcript]. Retrieved from http://www.nytimes.com/2008/01/01/health/nutrition/01chil.html_r=1&scp=90&sq=obesityst=nyt.

Barron, J. (2008, August 17). Restaurants must post calories, judge affirms. *New York Times* [archived web transcript]. Retrieved from http://www.nytimes.com/2008/04/17/nyregion/17calorie.html?_r=1&scp=99&sq=obesity&st=nyt.

Barry, C.L., Brescoll, V.L., Brownell, K.D. & Schlesinger, M. (2009). Obesity metaphors: How beliefs about the causes of obesity affect support for public policy. *The Milbank Quarterly*, *87*, 7–47.

Begley, S. (2009, January 17). The sins of the fathers, take two. *Newsweek* [archived web transcript]. Retrieved from http://www.newsweek.com/id/180103.

Brownell, K. (2009, February 1). Is it true that lack of sleep might lead to weight gain? *ABC News* [archived web transcript]. Retrieved from http://abcnews.go.com/Health/WellnessResource/story?id=6762328.

Campo, S. & Mastin, T. (2007). Placing the burden on the individual: Overweight and obesity in African-American and mainstream women's magazines. *Health Communication*, *23*, 229–240.

Carmichael, M. (2008a, August 24). Is there a surgical cure for diabetes? *Newsweek* [archived web transcript]. Retrieved from http://www.newsweek.com/2008/08/24/is-there-a-surgical-cure-for-diabetes.html.

Carmichael, M. (2008b, December 18). How fat went global. *Newsweek* [archived web transcript]. Retrieved from http://www.newsweek.com/id/175954.

Cloud, J. (2008, December 26). Nanny-state food regulations. *Time* [archived web transcript]. Retrieved from http://www.time.com/time/specials/2008/top10/article/0,30583,1855948_1864255_1864257,00.html.

Cloud, J. (2009, August 9). Why exercise won't make you thin. *Time* [archived web transcript]. Retrieved from http://www.time.com/time/health/article/0,8599,1914857-1,00.html.

Connolly-Ahern, C. & Broadway, S.C. (2008). 'To booze or not to booze?': Newspaper coverage of fetal alcohol spectrum disorders. *Science Communication*, *29*, 362–385.

Cooper, B. & Pease, E.C. (2008). The Mormons versus the 'Armies of Satan': Competing frames of morality in the *Brokeback Mountain* controversy in Utah newspapers. *Western Journal of Communication*, *73*, 134–156.

Crawford, R. (1980). Healthism and the medicalisation of everyday life. *International Journal of Health Services: Planning, Administration, Evaluation*, *10(3)*, 365–388.

Cruz, G. (2008, December 4). Why media could be bad for your child's health. *Time* [archived web transcript]. Retrieved from http://www.time.com/time/health/article/0,8599,1864141,00.html.

'Curb those cravings' (2009, May 10). Good Morning America, *ABC News* [LexisNexis web transcript]. Retrieved from http://www.lexisnexis.com.

Dutta, M.J. (2007). Communication about culture and health: Theorising culture-centred and cultural sensitivity approaches. *Communication Theory*, *17*, 304–328.

Entman, R. (1991). Framing U.S. coverage of international news: Contrasts in narratives of the KAL and Iran Air incidents. *Journal of Communication, 41(4)*, 6–27.

Entman, R.M. (1993). Framing: Toward clarification of a fractured paradigm. *Journal of Communication, 43(4)*, 51–58.

'Eye catching ads promote junk food to kids' (2008, July 29). CBS news [archived news transcript]. Retrieved from http://www.cbsnews.com/stories/2008/07/29/business/main4302213.shtml?tag=contentMain;contentBody.

Ferris, J. (2003). Parallel discourses and 'appropriate' bodies: Media constructions of anorexia and obesity in the cases of Tracey Gold and Carnie Wilson. *Journal of Communication Inquiry, 27*, 256–273.

Finkelstein, E.A. & Zuckerman, L. (2008). *The fattening of America: How the economy makes us fat, if it matters, and what to do about it.* Hoboken, NJ: Wiley & Sons.

'Food ads on Nickelodeon slammed in report' (2009, November 24). CBS News [archived web transcript]. Retrieved from http://www.cbsnews.com/stories/2009/11/24/health/healthy_living/main5761832.shtml?tag=contentMain;contentBody.

Fortin, J. (2009, January 22). Sugar free school. CNN [archived news video]. Retrieved from http://www.cnn.com/video/#/video/health/2009/01/22/fortin.hm.sugar.free.zone.cnn?iref=videosearch.

Fox, N.J. (1993). *Postmodernism, sociology, and health.* Buckingham: Open University Press.

Gard, M. & Wright, J. (2005). *The obesity epidemic: Science, morality, and technology*. New York: Routledge.

Gitlin, T. (1980). *The whole world is watching: Mass media in the making and unmaking of the New Left*. Berkeley: University of California Press.

Grumman, R. (2009, September 18) Why we eat too much. CNN Health [archived web transcript]. Retrieved from http://www.cnn.com/2009/HEALTH/09/18/why.overeat.eat.much/index.html?iref=allsearch.

Gupta, S. (2008a, June 9). Body of knowledge: Obesity. CNN [archived web transcript]. Retrieved from http://www.cnn.com/video/#/video/health/2008/06/09/bok.sensitivity.suit.cnn?iref=videosearch.

Gupta, S. (2008b, December 6). Fed up: America's killer diet. CNN [LexisNexis transcript]. Retrieved from http://www.lexisnexis.com.

Guttman, N. & Ressler, W.H. (2001). On being responsible: Ethical issues in appeals to personal responsibility in health campaigns. *Journal of Health Communication, 6*, 117–136.

Hallahan, K. (1999). Seven models of framing: Implications for public relations. *Journal of Public Relations Research, 11(3)*, 205–242.

'Health, United States' (2006). Centers for Disease Control and Prevention.

Heisley, M. (2008, September 8) Got a fat gene? Get active for 3–4 hours a day. *USA Today* [archived web transcript]. Retrieved from http://www.usatoday.com/news/health/weightloss/2008-09-08-obesity-gene_n.htm.

Hellmich, N. (2008, July 2). Restaurants as obesity cops doesn't sit well. *USA Today* [archived web transcript]. Retrieved from http://www.usatoday.com/news/health/2008-02-05-obesity-restaurant-law_n.htm.

Hellmich, N. (2009, January 7). Help kids maintain a healthy diet without a hefty cost. *USA Today* [archived web transcript]. Retrieved from http://www.usatoday.com/news/health/weightloss/2009-01-06-kids-diet_n.htm.

Horovitz, B. (2008, December 19). Schools takes steps to give kids more fruits, vegetables at lunch. *USA Today* [archived web transcript]. Retrieved from http://www.usatoday.com/moneyindustries/food/2008-12-17-kids-food-veggies-fruit_n.htm.

'How fat can be healthy' (2009, January 12). *Good Morning America*. ABC News [Lexis Nexis transcript]. Retrieved from http://www.lexisnexis.com.

'Irregular sleeping linked to obesity' (2009, May 7). *USA Today* [archived web transcript]. Retrieved from http://www.usatoday.com/news/health/2008-05-07-sleep-obesity_n.htm.

Iyengar, S. (1991). *Is anyone responsible? How television frames political issues*. Chicago: University of Chicago Press.

Johnston, H. (1995). A methodology for frame analysis: From discourse to cognitive schemata. In H. Johnston and B. Klandermans (eds), *Social movements and culture: Social movements, protest, and contention Volume 4* (pp. 217–246). Minneapolis, MN: University of Minnesota Press.

Judson, O. (2008, August 10). Honey, I plumped the kids. *New York Times* [Lexis Nexis Transcript]. Retrieved from http://www.lexisnexis.com.

Kantrowitz, B. & Wingert, P. (2008, July 8). What works. *Newsweek* [archived web transcript]. Retrieved from http://www.newsweek.com/id/144958.

Kersh, R. (2009). The Politics of Obesity. *Milbank Quarterly*, *87*, 295–316.

Kim, S. & Willis, L.A. (2007). Talking about obesity: News framing of who is responsible for causing and fixing the problem. *Journal of Health Communication*, *12*, 359–376.

Kingsbury, B. (2008, June 12). Fit at any size. *Time* [archived web transcript]. Retrieved from http://www.time.com/time/magazine/article/0,9171,1813993-1,00.html.

Kirkwood, W.G. & Brown, D. (1995). Public communication about the causes of disease: The rhetoric of responsibility. *Journal of Communication*, *45*, 55–76.

Kliff, S. (2008, October 16). The pleasure factor. *Newsweek* [archived web transcript]. Retrieved from http://www.newsweek.com/id/164197.

Kline, K.N. (2003). Popular media and health: Images, effects, and institutions. In T.L. Thompson, A.M. Dorsey, K.I. Miller & R. Parrott (eds), *Handbook of Health Communication* (pp. 557–581). Mahwah, NJ: Lawrence Erlbaum Associates.

Kluger, J. (2008, June 12). How America's children packed on the pounds. *Time* [archived web transcript]. Retrieved from http://www.time.com/time/health/article/0,8599,1813700,00.html.

'L.A. Council Poised to Ban Fast Food in Poor Neighbourhood' (2008, July 29). *USA Today* [archived web transcript]. Retrieved from http://www.usatoday.com/news/nation/2008-07-29-los-angeles-fast-food_n.htm.

Landau, E. (2009, October 24). Obesity, STDs flow in social networks. CNN [archived news transcript]. Retrieved from http://www.cnn.com/2009/TECH/10/24/tech.networks.connected/index.html?iref=allsearch.

Lawrence, R. (2004). Framing obesity: The evolution of news discourse on a public health issue. *The Harvard International Journal of Press/Politics*, *9*, 56–75.

Layton, L. (2009, April 27). Crave man. *Washington Post* [archived transcript, Lexis Nexis]. Retrieved from http://www.lexisnexis.com.

LeBesco, K. (2004). *Revolting bodies? The struggle to redefine fat identity*. Amherst, MA: University of Massachusetts.

Levy-Navarro, E. (2008). *The culture of obesity in early and late modernity*. New York: Palgrave Macmillan.

Losh, J. (2008, August 8). Dear parents: Your child is fat. *Time* [archived web transcript]. Retrieved from http://www.time.com/time/health/article/0,8599,1830796,00.html.

Lupton, D. (1994). *Medicine as culture: Illness, disease, and the body in Western societies*. London: Sage.

Lupton, D. (1995). *The imperative of health: Public health and the regulated body*. London: Sage.

Luther, C.A. & Zhou, X. (2005). Within the boundaries of politics: News framing of SARS in China and the United States. *Journalism & Mass Communication Quarterly*, *82*, 857–872.

Luu, E. (2009, October 9). Cookies, cakes, anything Mommy bakes banned at school. NBC News [archived news transcript]. Retrieved from http://www.nbcnewyork.com/news/health/Cookies-Cake-Anything-Mommy-Bakes-Banned-At-School-63853297.html.

Major, L.H. (2009). Break it to me harshly: The effects of intersecting news frames in lung cancer and obesity coverage. *Journal of Health Communication*, *14*, 174–188.

McInerney, F. (2006). Heroic frames: Discursive constructions around the requested death movement in Australia in the late 1990s. *Social Science & Medicine*, *62*, 654–667.

Mechanic, D. (2002). Disadvantage, inequality, and social policy: Major initiatives intended to improve population health may also increase health disparities. *Health Affairs*, *21*, 48–59.

Medina, J. (2009, October 2). A crackdown on bake sales in city schools. *New York Times* [archived web transcript]. Retrieved from http://www.nytimes.com/2009/10/03/nyregion/03bakesale.html.

Menashe, C.L. & Siegel, M. (1998). The power of a frame: Analysis of newspaper coverage of tobacco issues, United States, 1985–1996. *Journal of Health Communication*, *3*, 307–325.

Mindlin, A. (2008, Dec 24). The battle over the greens. *New York Times* [archived web transcript].http://www.nytimes.com/2008/02/24/nyregion/thecity/24cart.html?scp=8&sq=produce+carts&st=nyt.
Nagourney, E. (2008, September 22). Nutrition: Soda bans in schools has little impact. *New York Times* [archived web transcript]. Retrieved from http://www.nytimes.com/2008/09/23/health/nutrition/23nutr.html?scp=76&sq=obesity&st=nyt.
Nestle, M. (2002). *Food politics: How the food industry influence nutrition and health.* Berkeley: University of California.
'Obese Enjoy Eating Food Less and Less' (2008, October 20). CBS News [archived web transcript]. Retrieved from http://www.cbsnews.com/stories/2008/10/17/health/webmd/main4528147.shtml?tag=mncol;lst;3.
'Obesity and Overweight' (2006, September). World Health Organisation. Retrieved from http://www.who.int/mediacentre/factsheets/fs311/en/index.html.
'Obesity Bigger Threat Than Terrorism?' (2006, March 1). CBS News Online. Retrieved from http://www.cbsnews.com/stories/2006/03/01/health/main1361849.shtml.
Oliwenstein, L. (2008, June 12). Weighty issues for parents. *Time* [archived web transcript]. Retrieved from http://www.time.com/time/magazine/article/0,9171,1813953,00.html.
Park, A. (2008, September 8). Losing weight: Can exercise trump genes? *Time* [archived web transcript]. Retrieved from http://www.time.com/time/health/article/0,8599,1839708,00.html.
Park, A. (2009a, February 10). Mother's obesity raises risks of birth defects. *Time* [archived web transcript]. Retrieved from http://www.time.com/time/health/article/0,8599,1878549,00.html.
Park, A. (2009b, November 12). Another cause of obesity: The bacteria in your gut? *Time* [archived web transcript]. Retrieved from http://www.time.com/time/health/article/0,8599,1938023,00.html.
Parker-Pope, T. (2008, August 18). Better to be fat and fit than skinny and unfit. *New York Times* [archived web transcript]. Retrieved from http://www.nytimes.com/2008/08/19/health/19well.html?_r=2&scp=18&sq=obesity&st=nyt.
Peterson, A. & Lupton, D. (1996). *The new public health: Health and self in the age of risk.* London: Sage.
Powe, B.D., Daniels, E.C. & Finnie, R. (2005). Comparing perceptions of cancer fatalism among African American patients. *Journal of the American Academy of Nurse Practitioners*, *17*, 318–324.
Rabin, R.C. (2008, November 21). TV ads contribute to obesity, economists say. *New York Times* [archived web transcript]. Retrieved from http://www.nytimes.com/2008/11/21/health/research/21obesity.html?scp=3&sq=obesity&st=nyt.
Rabin, R.C. (2009a, June 9). Bad habits asserting themselves. *New York Times*, D:5.
Rabin, R.C. (2009b, December 15). New goal for the obese. *New York Times*, D:1.
Raymond, J. (2009, March 26). Big belly, bad memory. *Newsweek* [archived web transcript]. Retrieved from http://www.newsweek.com/id/129147/page/1.

Reese, S. (2001). Prologue – Framing public life: A bridging model for media research. In S. Reese, O. Gandy, & A. Grant (eds), *Framing public life: Perspectives on media and our understanding of the social world* (pp. 7–31). Mahwah, NJ: Lawrence Erlbaum.

'Restaurants fight NYC calories-on-menu law' (2008, June 22). *USA Today* [archived web transcript]. Retrieved from http://www.usatoday.com/news/health/weightloss/2008-04-22-nyc-menu_n.htm.

Rivera, R. (2008, August 28). Council vote for good health may weaken business at groceries in poor neighbourhoods. *New York Times* [archived web transcript]. Retrieved from http://www.nytimes.com/2008/02/28/nyregion/28grocer.html?_r=1&scp=98&sq=obesity&st=nyt.

Rochman, B. (2009, July 6). First comes love, then comes obesity? *Time* [archived web transcript]. Retrieved from http://www.time.com/time/magazine/article/0,9171,1907143,00.html.

Saguy, A.C. & Almeling, R. (2008). Fat in the fire? Science, the news media, and the 'obesity epidemic'. *Sociological Forum*, *23*, 53–83.

Salmon, C.T. (1989). Campaign for social improvement: An overview of values, rationales, and impacts. In C.T. Salmon (ed.), *Information campaign: Balancing social values and social change* (pp. 19–53). Newbury Park, CA: Sage.

St. George, D. (2008, December 2). Media bombardment linked to ill effects during childhood. *Washington Post* [archived web transcript]. Retrieved from http://www.washingtonpost.com/wp-dyn/content/article/2008/12/01/AR2008120102920.html.

Scheufele, D.A. (1999). Framing as a theory of media effects. *Journal of Communication*, *29*, 103–123.

Scheufele, D.A. (2000). Agenda-setting, priming, and framing revisited: Another look at cognitive effects of political communication. *Mass Communication & Society*, *3*, 297–316.

Schmitz, M.F., Filippone, P. & Edelman, E.M. (2003). Social representations of attention deficit/hyperactivity disorder. *Culture & Psychology*, *9*, 383–406.

Schneider, H. (2008, September 9). Report shows why it's smart to get your belly dancing. *Washington Post* [LexisNexis database]. Retrieved from http://www.lexisnexis.com.

Schwarz, H. (1986). *Never satisfied: A cultural history of diets, fantasies, and fat.* New York: Free Press.

Shaw, R.L. & Giles, D.C. (2009). Motherhood on ice? A media framing analysis of older mothers in the UK news. *Psychology & Health*, *24*, 221–236.

Shen, L., Condit, C.M. & Wright, L. (2009). The psychometric property and validation of a fatalism scale. *Psychology & Health*, 24, 597–613.

Shih, T.-J., Wijaya, R. & Brossard, D. (2008). Media coverage of public health epidemics: Linking framing and issue attention cycle toward an integrated theory of print. *Mass Communication and Society*, *11*, 141–160.

Shugart, H.A. (2010). Consuming citizen: Neoliberating the obese body. *Communication, Culture, and Critique*, *3(1)*, 105–126.

Signiorelli, N. (1993). *Mass media images and impact on health*. Westport, CT: Greenwood.

Sobal, J. & Maurer, D. (eds) (1999). *Weighty issues: Fatness and thinness as social problems*. New York: Aldine de Greuter.

Springen, K. (2008, November 7). Six facts about belly fat. *Newsweek* [archived web transcript]. Retrieved from http://www.newsweek.com/id/168129.

'Start Saying Goodbye to Belly Fat' (2008, November 1). *The Early Show*. New York: CBS Interactive [archived web transcript]. Retrieved from http://www.cbsnews.com/stories/2008/11/01/earlyshow/health/main4562801.shtml?tag=contentMain;contentBody.

Stein, R. (2009, December 17). Research links obesity to bacteria in digestive tract. *Washington Post* [archived web transcript]. Retrieved from http://www.washingtonpost.com/wpdyn/content/article/2009/12/20/AR2006122001271.html.

Stengel, R. (2008, June 12). A full plate. *Time* [archived web transcript]. Retrieved from http://www.time.com/time/magazine/article/0,9171,1813973,00.html.

'Study: Kids with obesity-linked gene drawn to fattening foods' (2008, December 12). *USA Today* [archived web transcript]. Retrieved from http://www.usatoday.com/news/health/weightloss/2008-12-12-obesity-gene_n.htm.

Summers, N. (2009, April 24). The economics of eating. *Newsweek* [archived web transcript]. Retrieved from http://search.newsweek.com/search?q=obesity+and+summers.

Szabo, L. (2008, December 2). Report: TV, internet harm kids. *USA Today* [archived web transcript]. Retrieved from http://www.usatoday.com/news/health/2008-12-01-media_N.htm?csp=34.

Tesh, S. (1994). Hidden arguments: Politics, ideology and disease prevention policy. New Brunswick: Rutgers University Press.

Waitzkin, H. (1991). *The politics of medical encounters*. New Haven: Yale University Press.

Wallack, L., Dorfman, L., Jernigan, D. & Themba, M. (1993). *Media advocacy and public health*. Newbury Park, CA: Sage.

Wallis, P. & Nerlich, B. (2005). Disease metaphors in new epidemics: The UK media framing of the 2003 SARS epidemic. *Social Science & Medicine*, *60*, 2629–2639.

Walsh, B. (2008, June 12). It's not just genetics. *Time* [archived web transcript]. Retrieved from http://www.time.com/time/magazine/article/0,9171,1813984,00.html.

Wingert, P. & Kantrowitz, B. (2009, May 28). Double trouble. *Newsweek* [archived web transcript]. Retrieved from http://www.newsweek.com/id/139031/page/1.

Wu, M. (2006). Framing AIDS in China: A comparative analysis of US and Chinese wire news coverage of HIV/AIDS in China. *Asian Journal of Communication*, *16*, 251–272.

Zoller, H.M. (2008). Technologies of neoliberal governmentality: The discursive influence of global economic policies in public health. In H.M. Zoller &

M.J. Dutta (eds), *Emerging perspectives in health communication: Meaning, culture, and power* (pp. 390–410). New York: Routledge.

Zoller, H.M. & Dutta, M.J. (2008). *Emerging perspectives in health communication: Meaning, culture, and power.* New York: Routledge.

Zoller, H.M. & Kline, K.N. (2008). Theoretical contributions of interpretive and critical research in health communication. *Communication Yearbook*, 32.

Index

Lightning Source UK Ltd.
Milton Keynes UK
UKOW06n2033121016

285148UK00014B/180/P